Library of
Davidson College

DEVELOPMENTAL STAGES IN HUMAN EMBRYOS

Including a Survey of the Carnegie Collection

Part A: Embryos of the First Three Weeks
(Stages 1 to 9)

RONAN O'RAHILLY

Department of Embryology
Carnegie Institution of Washington
Baltimore, Maryland

and

Department of Anatomy
Wayne State University School of Medicine
Detroit, Michigan

CARNEGIE INSTITUTION OF WASHINGTON
PUBLICATION 631

CARNEGIE INSTITUTION OF WASHINGTON
1530 P Street, N.W., Washington, D.C. 20005

COPYRIGHT © 1973 BY CARNEGIE INSTITUTION OF WASHINGTON

International Standard Book Number 0-87279-642-6
Library of Congress Catalog Card Number 73-84115

... the heart appears, like a speck of blood ...
*A little afterwards the body is differentiated,
at first very small and white*
      ARISTOTLE, *Historia Animalium*, 561a

PREFACE

For the past fifteen years the writer has had the privilege of studying the Carnegie Embryological Collection and of publishing research based on it. In December 1966 Dr. James D. Ebert, Director of the Department of Embryology, Carnegie Institution of Washington, invited the writer to continue and amplify the late Dr. Streeter's contributions on "Developmental Horizons in Human Embryos" and also to supplement and revise those already published. As a matter of practical convenience, these two functions have resulted in the division of the present work into two portions. Part A, which is being issued first, comprises the prenatal period up to three weeks (stages 1 to 9), that is, the phase of development not described by Dr. Streeter. Part B, to be issued subsequently and to be combined with Part A into one volume, will include the prenatal period from 3 to 8 weeks (stages 10 to 23). When the entire work becomes available, the artificial division into Parts A and B will disappear, and the human embryo will be considered during the first eight weeks of development.

At the present time, when such techniques as histochemistry and electron microscopy are already being applied in the study of human development, it seems particularly opportune to provide a detailed morphological account of the human embryo. The objectives of this monograph are basically those of Dr. George L. Streeter, as expressed by Dr. George W. Corner (1951), namely, to provide a descriptive atlas and bibliography of early human embryology, a formal classification by stages of embryonic development, a catalogue of the embryos in the Carnegie Collection, and a reference guide to important specimens in other laboratories.

It is hoped that the Carnegie staging system will be accepted and used internationally, thereby allowing detailed comparisons to be made between the findings at one institution and those at another.

That the very early stages of human development can now be described is due in no small measure to the presence in the Carnegie Collection of specimens donated by Drs. Hertig and Rock. Prepared with the aid of the late Dr. Heuser's technical skill, these embryos have yet to be surpassed in excellence and rarity.

During the past two years this undertaking has been supported in part by the U. S. National Institutes of Health General Research Support Grant, Wayne State University. The writer wishes to take this occasion to acknowledge also the willing assistance that he has received over the years from the research members and from the technical and clerical staff of the Carnegie Department of Embryology. Most of the drawings in the present work were prepared in the Department of Art as Applied to Medicine, the Johns Hopkins School of Medicine, under the direction of Mrs. Ranice Crosby, and thanks are due to Mrs. Marjorie Gregerman, Mrs. Diane Abeloff, and Mrs. Barbara Grossman of that department. The ready assistance and interest of Miss Nancy Kolzak, Smith College, in the arranging and cataloguing of the collection have been of considerable aid. Dr. Elizabeth M. Ramsey, Carnegie Institution, and Dr. Theodore W. Torrey, Professor of Zoology, Indiana University, have kindly read the original typescript and have made a number of valuable suggestions. It is a particular pleasure to thank Dr. Ramsey and Professor Ebert for their continued encouragement, advice, and friendship during the preparation of this monograph.

In conclusion, the great care exercised by Miss Sheila McGough, Editor, and the publication staff of the Carnegie Institution during the preparation of the text and illustrations for publication is greatly appreciated.

CONTENTS

Introduction 1

Stage 1 9

Stage 2 15

Stage 3 23

Stage 4 29

Stage 5 33

Stage 6 59

Stage 7 83

Stage 8 103

Stage 9 123

Concluding Remark 143

References 149

Specimen Index 161

Index 165

INTRODUCTION

*The norm should be established;
embryos should be arranged in stages.*

FRANKLIN P. MALL

The combined use of fixation, sectioning with a microtome, and reconstruction from the resultant sections first enabled Wilhelm His, senior, to begin to elucidate thoroughly the anatomy of individual human embryos.

Although fixatives other than spirits were introduced early in the nineteenth century, formalin was not employed until the 1890s. His devised a microtome in about 1866. (A microtome had already been employed as early as 1770.) The wax plate reconstruction technique of Born (1883), introduced in 1876, has undergone numerous modifications over the years. These, as well as graphic reconstruction, have been discussed in a number of publications, e.g., by Gaunt (1971). Florian, who used graphic reconstruction of the human embryo to great advantage, elaborated the mathematical background in Czech in 1928. (See also Fetzer and Florian, 1930.)

It has been pointed out that "the idea of working out a complete account of the development of the human body was always before the mind of His" (Keibel and Mall, 1910), and his collaborator, Franz Keibel, proposed to provide "an account of the development of the human body, based throughout on human material" (*ibid.*) rather than from the comparative standpoint. The result was the *Manual of Human Embryology* edited by Keibel and Mall (1910, 1912), which was an important step in the goal of seeking precision in human embryology. The hope was expressed that, subsequently, a second attempt, "whether made by us or by others, will come so much nearer the goal" (*ibid.*).

The Carnegie Collection

Mall's collection of human embryos, begun in 1887, later became the basis of the Carnegie Collection (Mall and Meyer, 1921). Mall (1913) stated his indebtedness to His in the following terms: "We must thank His for the first attempt to study carefully the anatomy of human embryos, but his work was planned on so large a scale that he never completed it... Thus we may trace back to him the incentive for Keibel's *Normentafeln*, Minot's great collection of vertebrate embryos and mine of human embryos." In more recent years the Carnegie Collection has benefited enormously from the meticulous investigations of Bartelmez, the technical adroitness of Heuser, and the donation of, as well as research on, remarkably young specimens by Hertig and Rock. The microtomy of Messrs. Charles H. Miller and William H. Duncan, the reconstructions by Mr. Osborne O. Heard, the artwork by Mr. James F. Didusch, and the photography of Messrs. Chester F. Reather and Richard D. Grill, have each played a key role in the establishment of the superb embryological collection on which the present monograph is so largely based. In George W. Corner's apt comparison, the Collection serves "as a kind of Bureau of Standards."

Embryological Seriation

His had made the first thorough arrangement of human embryos in the form of a series of selected individual embryos, numbered in the presumed order of their development. The same principle was followed in the published plates known as the *Normentafeln* edited by Franz Keibel from 1897 onwards; the volume on the human (by Keibel and Elze) appeared in 1908. The limitations of the method are (1) that individual embryos cannot be arranged in a perfect series, because any given specimen may be advanced in one respect while being retarded in another; and (2) that it may prove impossible to match a new embryo exactly with any one of the illustrated norms. The need for a more flexible procedure than a mere *Entwicklungsreihe* soon became apparent in experimental embryology.

Embryonic Staging

In the words of Ross G. Harrison (Wilens, 1969), "the need for standardized stages in the embryonic development of various organisms for the purpose of accurate description of normal development and for utilization in experimental work has long been recognized." Because "development is a continuous process with an indefinite number of stages" (*ibid.*), a certain number have to be chosen. Thus each stage "is merely an arbitrarily cut section through the time-axis of the life of an organism" (deBeer, 1958). It resembles, in Harrison's apt comparison, a frame taken from a cine-film. Stages are based on the apparent morphological state of development, and hence are not directly dependent on either chronological age or on size. Furthermore, comparison is made of a number of features of each specimen, so that individual differences are rendered less significant and a certain latitude of variation is taken into account.

Although embryonic staging had been introduced towards the end of the nineteenth century, it was first employed in human embryology by Franklin P. Mall (1914), founder of the Department of Embryology of the Carnegie Institution of Washington.

On the basis of photographs of their external form, Mall (1914) arranged 266 human embryos from 2 to 25 mm in length in a series of 14 stages, lettered from H to U. (A to G were to have been the earlier stages.)

Mall's successor, George L. Streeter, provided the definitive classification of human embryos into stages, which he termed "developmental horizons." Attention was concentrated on embryos up to about 32 mm C.-R. (crown–rump) length because it was believed that, during the fetal period, the rate of increment in size and weight might be large enough to provide an adequate index of relative development.

The original plan was "to cover as far as possible the earliest specimens up to fetuses between 32 and 38 mm. long, the stage at which the eyelids have come together," and "twenty-five age groups" were envisioned (Streeter, 1942). Subsequently, Streeter (1951) decided that stage 23 "could be considered to mark the ending of the embryonic period" proper. The onset of marrow formation in the humerus was "arbitrarily adopted as the conclusion of the embryonic and the beginning of the fetal period of prenatal life. It occurs in specimens about 30 mm. in length" (Streeter, 1949). A scheme of the 23 stages, as modified and used in the present monograph, is provided in Table 1, and a comparison between the stages and the original "Developmental Horizons" is given in Table 2.

The term "horizon" was borrowed from geology and archaeology by Streeter (1942) in order "to emphasize the importance of thinking of the embryo as a

INTRODUCTION

TABLE 1. Developmental Stages in Human Embryos

Carnegie Stage	Pairs of Somites	Length (mm)	Age (days)[1]	Age (days)[2]	Features
1				1	Fertilization.
2			1½–3	2–3	From 2 to about 16 cells.
3			4	4–5	Free blastocyst.
4			5–6	5–6	Attaching blastocyst.
5		0.1–0.2	7–12	7–12	Implanted although previllous.
5a		0.1	7–8		Solid trophoblast.
5b		0.1	9		Trophoblastic lacunae.
5c		0.15–0.2	11–12		Lacunar vascular circle.
6		0.2	13	13–15	Chorionic villi; primitive streak may appear.
6a					Chorionic villi.
6b					Primitive streak.
7		0.4	16	15–17	Notochordal process.
8		1.0–1.5	18	17–19	Primitive pit; notochordal and neurenteric canals.
9	1–3	1.5–2.5	20	19–21	Somites first appear.
10	4–12	2–3.5	22	22–23	Neural folds begin to fuse; 2 pharyngeal bars; optic sulcus.
11	13–20	2.5–4.5	24	23–26	Rostral neuropore closes; optic vesicle.
12	21–29	3–5	26	26–30	Caudal neuropore closes; 3 pharyngeal bars; upper limb buds appearing.
13	30–?	4–6	28	28–32	Four limb buds; lens disc; otic vesicle.
14		5–7	32	31–35	Lens pit and optic cup; endolymphatic appendage distinct.
15		7–9	33	35–38	Lens vesicle; nasal pit; antitragus beginning; hand plate; trunk relatively wider; cerebral vesicles distinct.
16		8–11	37	37–42	Nasal pit faces ventrally; retinal pigment visible in intact embryo; auricular hillocks beginning; foot plate.
17		11–14	41	42–44	Head relatively larger; trunk straighter; nasofrontal groove distinct; auricular hillocks distinct; finger rays.
18		13–17	44	44–48	Body more cuboidal; elbow region and toe rays appearing; eyelids beginning; tip of nose distinct; nipples appear; ossification may begin.
19		16–18	47½	48–51	Trunk elongating and straightening.
20		18–22	50½	51–53	Upper limbs longer and bent at elbows.
21		22–24	52	53–54	Fingers longer; hands approach each other, feet likewise.
22		23–28	54	54–56	Eyelids and external ear more developed.
23		27–31	56½	56–60	Head more rounded; limbs longer and more developed.

[1] Olivier and Pineau (1962) for stages 11 to 23; miscellaneous sources for stages 1 to 10.
[2] Jirásek (1971).

living organism which in its time takes on many guises, always progressing from the smaller and simpler to the larger and more complex" (*ibid.*). However, the somewhat infelicitous term "horizon" is replaced here by "stage" because the latter is the simple term employed for all other vertebrate embryos. Not only was the term "stage" used decades ago by Harrison for *Ambystoma* and subsequently by Hamburger and Hamilton for the chick embryo, as well as by others for a variety of reptiles, birds, and mammals, but, even in the case of the human,

TABLE 2. Comparison between Present Staging System and Streeter's "Developmental Horizons."

Carnegie Stage	Streeter's (1942) Criteria	Developmental Horizon
1	Unicellular	I
2	Segmentation	II
3	Free blastocyst	III
4–5	Implanting	IV
5	Implanted but avillous	V
	Chorionic villi	VI
	Distinct yolk sac	
6	Branching villi	
	Axis of germ disc defined	VII
	Primitive groove	
	Primitive node	VIII
7	Notochordal process	
		IX
8	Neural folds	
9	1–3 pairs of somites	
10	4–12 pairs of somites	X
11	13–20 pairs of somites	XI
12	21–29 pairs of somites	XII

the term "stage" was employed by Mall (1914) when he first staged the human embryo more than half a century ago. The term is simpler, clearer, of widespread usage, and can be employed as a verb (to stage an embryo) as well as a participial adjective (a staging system). Furthermore, it should be pointed out that such expressions as "at the 3 mm stage" should be replaced by "at 3 mm." In other words, the length of an embryo is a single criterion that is not in itself sufficient to establish a stage. The term "stage" should be confined to its present-day usage in embryology (such as the 46 stages of Hamburger and Hamilton in the chick, and the 46 stages of Harrison in *Ambystoma maculatum*).

Additional alterations that have been made in the current work include the replacement of Roman by Arabic numerals and the elimination of the scientifically meaningless term "ovum."

Stages 10 to 23 were published either by Streeter (1942, 1945, 1948, and 1951) or at least with the aid of his notes (Heuser and Corner, 1957). "The earliest age groups" were wisely "to be reserved to the last, so that advantage may be taken of any new material that becomes available" (Streeter, 1942). These groups, stages 1 to 9, which were to have been completed by the late Dr. Chester H. Heuser, became the task of the present writer.

Embryonic Length

Because most embryos are received already in fixative, it is more practicable for comparisons to use measurement after fixation as the standard (Streeter, 1945). The most useful single measurement is the greatest length of the embryo as measured in a straight line (that is, caliper length) without any attempt to straighten the natural curvature of the specimen. Up to stage 10, measurements are frequently made on accurately scaled models, although the results (owing to shrinkage in preparing the sections) are then smaller (by 25 per cent, according to Streeter, 1942).[1]

The crown–rump (C.-R.) length appears to have been introduced into embryology by Arnold in 1887 (Keibel and Mall, 1910), although the sitting height had been used as a measurement in the adult by Leonardo da Vinci (McMurrich, 1930). In the human embryo, from about stage 12 onwards it becomes practicable to use the C.-R. instead of the greatest length, and this is usually done in the later stages. At first, owing to increasing

[1] A particularly interesting study has been made of the shrinkage of (pig) embryos in the procedures preparatory to sectioning (Patten and Philpott, 1921). Careful technique (see Heard, 1957) is naturally to be encouraged in order to keep artifactual changes to a minimum.

INTRODUCTION

curvature of the embryo, the C.-R. is less than the maximum length but, in the later stages of the embryonic period proper, the two lengths are basically equal. The C.-R. length, or sitting height, continues to be the most useful measurement in the fetal period, although other mensural criteria, such as foot length, may profitably be employed, particularly if the specimen has been damaged. The C.-R. length, which should always be stated in millimeters, is taken in a straight line according to the specifications laid down by Mall (1907), without disturbing the natural, curved posture of the embryo, and preferably (for purposes of standardization) after two weeks in 10 per cent formalin (Streeter, 1920). Particularly in the case of larger embryos and all fetuses, the C.-R. length of a given specimen should always be stated in preference to, or at least in addition to, its supposed age.

The embryonic lengths given in Table 1 indicate the suggested norms. Where possible they are based on specimens graded as excellent and after fixation. It should be stressed, however, that the figures do not indicate the full range within a given stage, especially when specimens of poor quality are included.

Body weight has been somewhat neglected within the embryonic period proper, although some data are available (Witschi, 1956a; Jirásek, Uher, and Uhrová, 1966; Nishimura et al. 1968). By stage 23, the embryo weighs about 2 to 2.7 grams.

Embryonic Age

The supposed age, as dubiously estimated from the menstrual history, is seldom useful within the embryonic period proper, and such expressions as "at the 18-day stage" should have no place in present-day embryology. Moreover, allowance should be made, but generally is not, for considerable variability in both premenstrual (Vollman, 1967) and postmenstrual (Stewart, 1952) phases of the menstrual cycle, as well as for the possibility of incorrect identification of menstruation or erroneous interpretation of its absence (Treloar, Behn, and Cowan, 1967).

The ages of very early human embryos (those of the first three or four weeks) have been estimated chiefly by comparing their development with that of monkey conceptuses of known postovulatory ages (Rock and Hertig, 1944). Coital history, the condition of the corpus luteum, and the appearance of the endometrium are also taken into account (Rock and Hertig, 1948). More recently, ovulation tests are providing additional information.

When an embryo has been staged, its presumed age in postovulatory days can be gauged from an appropriate table. The term "postovulatory age" (fig. 1) refers to the length of time since the last ovulation before pregnancy began. Because fertilization must occur very close to the time of ovulation, the postovulatory interval is a satisfactory indication of embryonic age. "Menstrual age," on the other hand, is a misnomer in that it does not indicate age.

In Table 1, two columns are devoted to age. In the first, that originally selected for this monograph, the ages are based on Hertig, Rock, and Adams (1956) for stages 2 to 7, on Heuser (1932) for stage 8, on Ludwig (1928) for stage 9, on Heuser and Corner (1957) for stage 10, and on Olivier and Pineau (1962) for stages 11 to 23.

The range is not indicated but (at least for stages 10 to 23) it was believed by Streeter to be ± 1 day for any given stage. It should be noted, however, that, from stage 14 onwards, the ages become

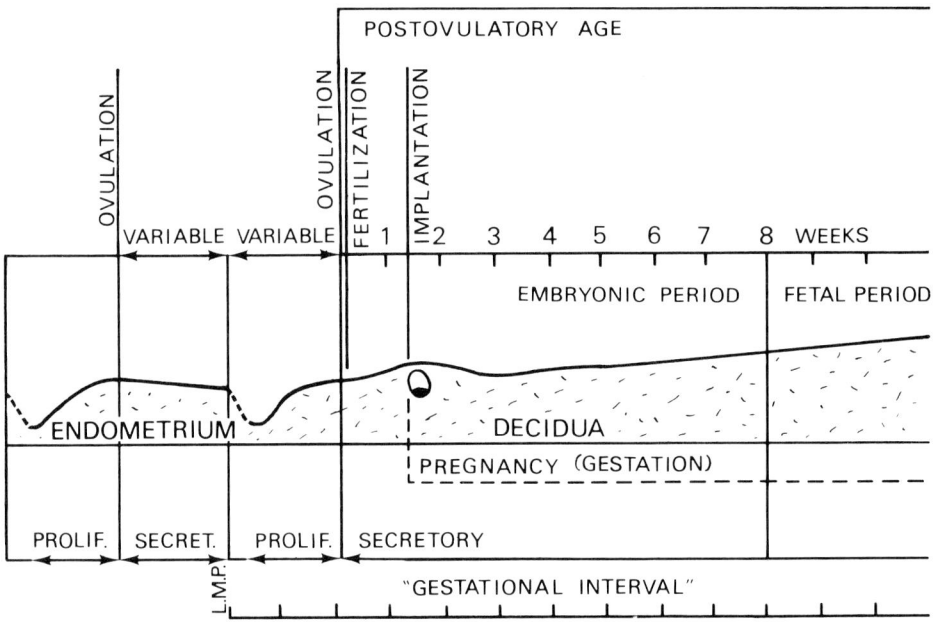

Fig. 1. Diagram of endometrial-decidual and embryonic-fetal relationships in relation to time. The second ovulation shown, which is followed by fertilization, is that from which postovulatory age is calculated. The last menstrual period (L.M.P.), which occurred a variable time previously, marks the beginning of the "gestation interval," as defined by Treloar, Behn, and Cowan (1967), who consider pregnancy (gestation) to begin with implantation. Postconceptual hemorrhage in phase with menstruation would result in an apparently short gestational interval. On the other hand, an unrecognized abortion preceding pregnancy, if no menstruation intervened, would result in an apparently long gestational interval. Such possibilities, together with variability in both premenstrual and postmenstrual phases of the cycle, render menstrual data unsatisfactory in the assessment of embryonic age.

increasingly greater than those given by Streeter, which were based on comparisons with macaque embryos; it is now known that such comparisons are not warranted at these stages. Thus, by the time that the embryo reaches stage 23, there is general agreement that it is not 47 ± 1 days (Streeter, 1951) but rather at least 56 days (Witschi, 1956a; Olivier and Pineau, 1962; Jirásek, Uher, and Uhrová, 1966; Jirásek, 1971).[2]

More recently, a table of "gestational age ... estimated from anamnestic data available for embryos in the author's collection" has been published by Jirásek (1971) and has been incorporated here as the second column of ages in Table 1. It is not without interest to note that, with but few exceptions (chiefly stage 15), the figures given by Jirásek resemble closely those provided by Olivier and Pineau. Although in a few instances (stages 17, 19, 20, and 21) Jirásek's ages are half to one day older, in most cases the figures of Olivier and Pineau fall within the range listed by Jirásek. With regard to the early stages, it should be pointed out that Jirásek used "Streeter's horizons" and hence his VI and VII, for example, both correspond to Carnegie stage 6, and his VIII corresponds more closely to Carnegie stage 7. To avoid further con-

[2] Other suggestions include "about 52 days" (Iffy et al., 1967) and "5 days more than Streeter's" age, hence also approximately 52 days (Nishimura et al., 1968).

INTRODUCTION

fusion, however, allowance for this has not been made in Table 1.

Alternative Systems of Staging

For the sake of completeness, it should be mentioned that two alternative systems of staging the human embryo have been published, although the use of each appears to have been restricted to its author.

Mazanec's (1953, 1959) scheme was limited to the period of development ("blastogenesis") from the oocyte up to (but not including) the first appearance of somites, as follows:

Group I. Oocytes
 II. Segmentation
 III. Abembryonic pole uncovered
 IV. Implanted
 V. Chorionic villi
 VI. Branching chorionic villi; primitive streak and node; cloacal membrane
 VII. Vascularization of chorion; notochordal process and canal

The corresponding stages are indicated in Table 3 for purposes of comparison, although, because the criteria are somewhat different, a precise equivalence is not possible.

Witschi's (1956a) scheme, which includes the entire period of prenatal life (although the fetal period is relegated to three stages), is based on the attractive idea of using a standard system of enumeration throughout vertebrate embryology (Witschi, 1956a, 1956b, 1962). Thus a vertebrate embryo that possesses from 13 to 20 pairs of somites, for example, would be classified as Witschi's stage 16. The difficulty, of course, is that such an embryo would under present conditions be classified as stages 28–32 if it were *Ambystoma maculatum*, as stages 11–13 if it were *Gallus domesticus*, and as stage 11 if it were *Homo sapiens*. To introduce a new scheme of numbering of stages into human embryology at this late moment, however, would run the risk of causing very considerable confusion, and it has not been deemed justifiable to make such an attempt in the present work.

Witschi's stages are listed in Table 3, where they are compared with the stages used in this monograph (and not with the original plan of Streeter's horizons, it should be noted). Thus, if Witschi's scheme were to receive the international approval that he had hoped for, Table 3 would permit the appropriate substitutions to be made in the present work.

TABLE 3. Comparison of Present Staging System and Those of Mazanec and Witschi

Carnegie Stage	Mazanec's Group	Witschi's Stage
1	I	1
2	} II	2–4
3		5–6
4	. . .	7
5		8–10
5a	} III	
5b		
5c	IV	
6		11
6a	V	
6b	VI	
7	} VII	
8		. . .
9		12–13
10		14
11		14–15
12		16
13		17–19
14		20–24
15		25
16		26
17		27
18		28–29
19		30–31
20		32
21		}33
22		
23		34
Fetal period		34–36

Indeed, such flexibility is a characteristic of a well-designed staging system. The interpretation of what constitutes a 41-day human embryo, for example, not only may change but actually has changed over the past two decades, whereas the defining characters of a stage-17 embryo have remained intact.

It should be pointed out that the criteria used by Hendrickx (1971) for staging the baboon differ in a number of small but important respects from those employed here for the human, and hence great caution should be exercised in making comparisons.

Normality

The majority of the approximately 600 sectioned Carnegie embryos assigned to the 23 stages are listed as normal, although variations in, and even anomalies of, individual organs are probably not uncommon. At least 100 out of more than 200 embryos, for example, have recently been reported to show some degree of neuroschisis (Padget, 1970). It should not be assumed, however, that every minor defect would necessarily lead to a recognizable anomaly in later life. In the present investigation, an effort has been made to eliminate, or at least to note specifically, the presence of frankly abnormal specimens. Nevertheless, it is still true that "as our knowledge of the normal becomes more complete, we find that more and more young embryos which formerly were regarded as normal are not really so . . . it remains impossible even at the present time, to determine in all cases whether we are dealing with a normal or an abnormal specimen, even after it has been mounted in serial sections" (Meyer in Mall and Meyer, 1921). It may be concluded that "The Borderland of Embryology and Pathology" (Willis, 1962) continues to be an important and fruitful area of investigation.

STAGE 1

Embryonic life commences with fertilization [1] and hence the beginning of fertilization may be taken as the *point de départ* of stage 1.

Fertilization is the procession of events that begins when a spermatozoon makes contact with an oocyte or its investments and ends with the intermingling of maternal and paternal chromosomes at metaphase of the first mitotic division of the zygote (Brackett *et al.*, 1972). Fertilization requires probably slightly longer than 24 hours in primates (*ibid.*). In the case of human oocytes fertilized *in vitro*, pronuclei were formed within 11 hours of insemination (Edwards, 1972).

Fertilization, which takes place normally in the ampulla of the uterine tube, includes (a) contact of spermatozoa with the zona pellucida of an oocyte, penetration of one or more spermatozoa through the zona pellucida and the ooplasm, swelling of the spermatozoal head and extrusion of the second polar body; (b) the formation of the male and female pronuclei; and (c) the beginning of the first mitotic division, or cleavage, of the zygote.[2] The various details of fertilization, including such matters as criteria, capacitation, acrosome reaction, and activation, should be sought in special works (e.g., that edited by Moghissi and Hafez, 1972).

The three phases (a, b, and c) referred to above will be included here under stage 1, the characteristic feature of which is unicellularity. The sequence of events before and during the first three stages is summarized in Table 4.

The term "ovum," which has been used for such disparate structures as an oocyte and a three-week embryo, has no scientific usefulness and is avoided here; the term "egg" is best reserved for a nutritive object frequently seen on the breakfast table.

At ovulation, the oocyte is a large cell surrounded by a thick covering, the zona pellucida, which is believed to be produced (at least largely) by the surrounding follicular cells. Processes of the follicular cells and microvilli of the oocyte both extend into the zona. The diameter of such a mammalian cell, including its zona, ranges from 70 to 190 micrometers. In the human, the ooplasm measures about 95, and the thickness of the zona ranges from 12 to 18 micrometers (Allen

---

[1] Despite the small size (*ca.* 0.1 mm) and weight (*ca.* 0.004 mg) of the organism at fertilization, "ist sie schon ein individual-spezifischer Mensch..." (Blechschmidt, 1972). The complexity of the possible implications of this should not be underestimated (Dedek, 1972). According to Treloar, Behn, and Cowan (1967), "the initiation of a new life" occurs at that moment when fertilization "is completed by fusion of the two sets of chromosomes." Pregnancy, however, is considered by these authors to be established when the blastocyst "is durably implanted in the uterine mucosa." Thus, on this basis, pregnancy (gestation) would be shorter than postovulatory age, which is in turn shorter than "gestational interval" (from the onset of the last menstrual period to the time of birth).

[2] In a study of the ewe, cow, and rabbit, Thibault (1967) subdivided fertilization into the following five stages: (1) after passage through the corona radiata and zona pellucida ("stage 0"), the spermatozoon becomes anchored to the microvilli of the cytoplasmic membrane; (2) the spermatozoon penetrates the ooplasm, and the second polar body is formed; (3) the male and then the female pronucleus form; (4) the pronuclei approach each other, and the DNA becomes duplicated; and (5) the pronuclei unite (which has been denied; see later) and the first segmentation mitosis ensues.

TABLE 4. Tabulation of the First Three Stages

Stage	Event	Products
	1st meiotic division	
		Secondary oocyte and 1st polar body
	Beginning of 2nd meiotic division and ovulation	
		Ovulated oocyte
1a	Fertilization { Penetration	Penetrated oocyte
1b	Completion of 2nd meiotic division and formation of pronuclei	Ootid and 2nd polar body
	Pronuclei enter cleavage division	
1c		Zygote
	Cleavage continues	
2		2 to about 16 cells
	Formation of segmentation cavity	
3		Blastocyst, from about 32 cells onwards

et al., 1930). Excellent photomicrographs and electron micrographs of human secondary oocytes are available (e.g., Baca and Zamboni, 1967, figs. 20 to 24; Kennedy and Donahue, 1969). The zona pellucida is covered externally by the corona radiata, which is a loose investment of granulosa cells from the ovarian follicle. On fixation and embedding, the oocyte of the pig "undergoes a shrinkage of about 40 per cent" and this affects the cytoplasm more than the zona (Heuser and Streeter, 1929), so that a subzonal (or perivitelline) space becomes accentuated. The polar bodies are found within that space. It is said that the first polar body may divide before the second is released, and it has been claimed that each of the three polar bodies is capable of being fertilized (Shettles, 1958). Although it is not unusual for the second polar body to display a nucleus, the chromosomes of the first polar body are isolated and naked (Zamboni, 1971).

It is "likely that no more than one day intervenes between ovulation and fertilization. This time interval may be taken then as the possible error in age of [an] embryo when it is considered the same as ovulatory age" (Rock and Hertig, 1942).

(a) Penetrated oocyte. What are believed to be penetrated oocytes have been seen in certain mammals, e.g., in the hamster (Hamilton and Samuel, 1956) and, with the aid of electron microscopy, in the rabbit (Hadek, 1969) and the mouse (Zamboni, 1971, 1972). In the human, in oocytes matured *in vitro* and subjected to insemination *in vitro*, the occurrence of spermatozoal penetration has been inferred from the presence of spermatozoa in the zona pellucida or in the subzonal space (Edwards, Bavister, and Steptoe, 1969). In strict usage, however, the term "penetrated oocyte" should be employed only "after gamete plasma membranes have become confluent" (Zamboni *et al.*, 1966).

(b) Ootid. The cell characterized by the presence of the male and female pronuclei is termed an ootid (figs. 2a, 2b, and 3). Several examples of human ootids have been described. They are

probably about 12 to 24 hours in age. The diameter, including the zona pellucida, is about 175 micrometers (Hamilton, 1946; Dickmann et al., 1965), and the diameter of the subzonal space is approximately 140. The cytoplasm of the ootid has a diameter of about 100 micrometers (Hamilton, 1946; Noyes et al., 1965); each of the pronuclei measures about 30 (Zamboni et al., 1966). The various ultrastructural features of the ootid have been described and illustrated in the case of the only specimen so far examined by electron microscopy (Zamboni et al., 1966).

Although, "in most mammalian species, the male pronucleus has been reported to be larger than the female pronucleus," the converse has been found in one human specimen and, in two others, the pronuclei appeared to be of equal size (Zamboni, 1971).

Two ootids (one described as "in syngamy," Hendrickx, 1971) have been described and illustrated in the baboon, *Papio sp.* (Hendrickx and Kraemer, 1968). Their diameters (including the zonae) were 178 and 155 micrometers, respectively, and they each included two polar bodies.

(c) Zygote. The cell that characterizes the last phase of fertilization is elusive. The first cleavage spindle forms rapidly and has been used in identification. Such cells have probably been seen in certain mammals, e.g., the pig (Heuser and Streeter, 1929), the cow (Hamilton and Laing, 1946), the hamster (Hamilton and Samuel, 1956), the rat (Schlafke and Enders, 1967), and the mouse (Zamboni, 1972).

On the basis of ultrastructural studies of the rabbit, "pronuclear fusion does not exist in the rabbit zygote." Rather, when the two pronuclear envelopes break down, "the two groups of chromosomes move together and assume positions on the first cleavage spindle. Thus, in the rabbit, there is an absence of a zygote nucleus" (Longo and Anderson, 1969). Indeed, the development of a fertilization nucleus resulting from the fusion (synkaryosis) of male and female pronuclei, a well-documented characteristic in the sea urchin, "does not occur in mammalian zygotes where the parental pronuclei enter prophase of the first cleavage division in an independent fashion" (Zamboni, 1971).

In the human, the initial cleavage that heralds the onset of stage 2 occurs in the uterine tube "some time between twenty-four and thirty hours after [the beginning of] fertilization" (Hertig, 1968).

SPECIMENS OF STAGE 1 ALREADY DESCRIBED

Ootids have been described by the following authors:

Hamilton (1946 and 1949). Tubal. Diameter (including zona pellucida), 173 micrometers. Diameter of ooplasm, 100 micrometers. Sectioned serially at 7 micrometers. Two pronuclei, one larger than the other. Many spermatozoa in zona pellucida. Dickmann et al. (1965) have expressed some doubts about this specimen.

Khvatov (1959). Tubal. Two pronuclei, claimed to be distinguished as male and female.

Dickmann et al. (1965). Tubal. Diameter (including zona), 174 micrometers. Zona pellucida, 17.5 micrometers in thickness. Diameter of ooplasm, 103 micrometers (Noyes et al. 1965). Two pronuclei, approximately equal in size (fig. 2b). Nucleoli visible. Tail of fertilizing spermatozoon identified over one pronucleus. Well illustrated (figs. 2a and 2b).

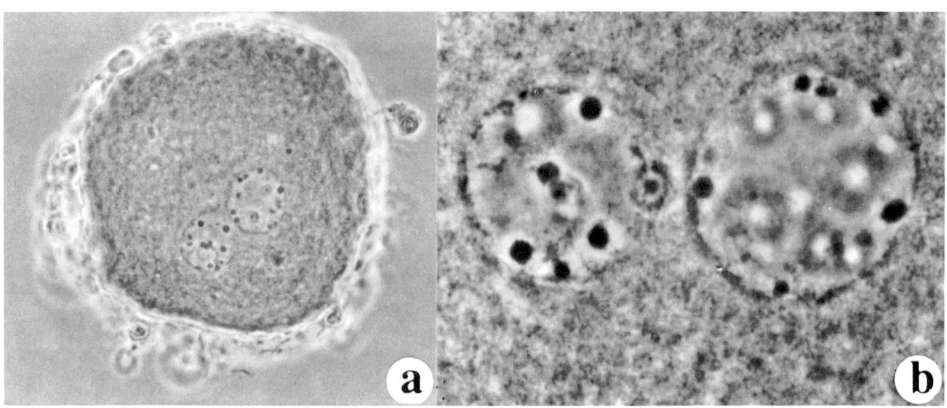

Fig. 2a. Phase contrast view of human ootid after fixation and staining. The zona pellucida has been dissolved during preparation of the specimen. By courtesy of Dr. Z. Dickmann and the *Anatomical Record*. b. Phase contrast, oil immersion view of the pronuclei shown in figure 2a. By courtesy of Dr. Z. Dickmann and the *Anatomical Record*.

Zamboni et al. (1966). Tubal. Ootid estimated to have a maximum diameter of about 150 micrometers, and 110 to 120 without the zona pellucida (Zamboni, personal communication, 1970). Fixed and sectioned for electron microscopy. Zona seen and 3 polar bodies identified. Two pronuclei, of about equal size (30 micrometers), each with a spheroidal nucleolus. Remnants of penetrating spermatozoon identified near one pronucleus. Ultrastructural findings described in detail and well illustrated (fig. 3).

Edwards, Bavister, and Steptoe (1969). Seven ootids resulted from insemination *in vitro* of oocytes matured *in vitro*. Two had two pronuclei each, four had three each, and one had five. Photographs, but no cytological details, were provided.

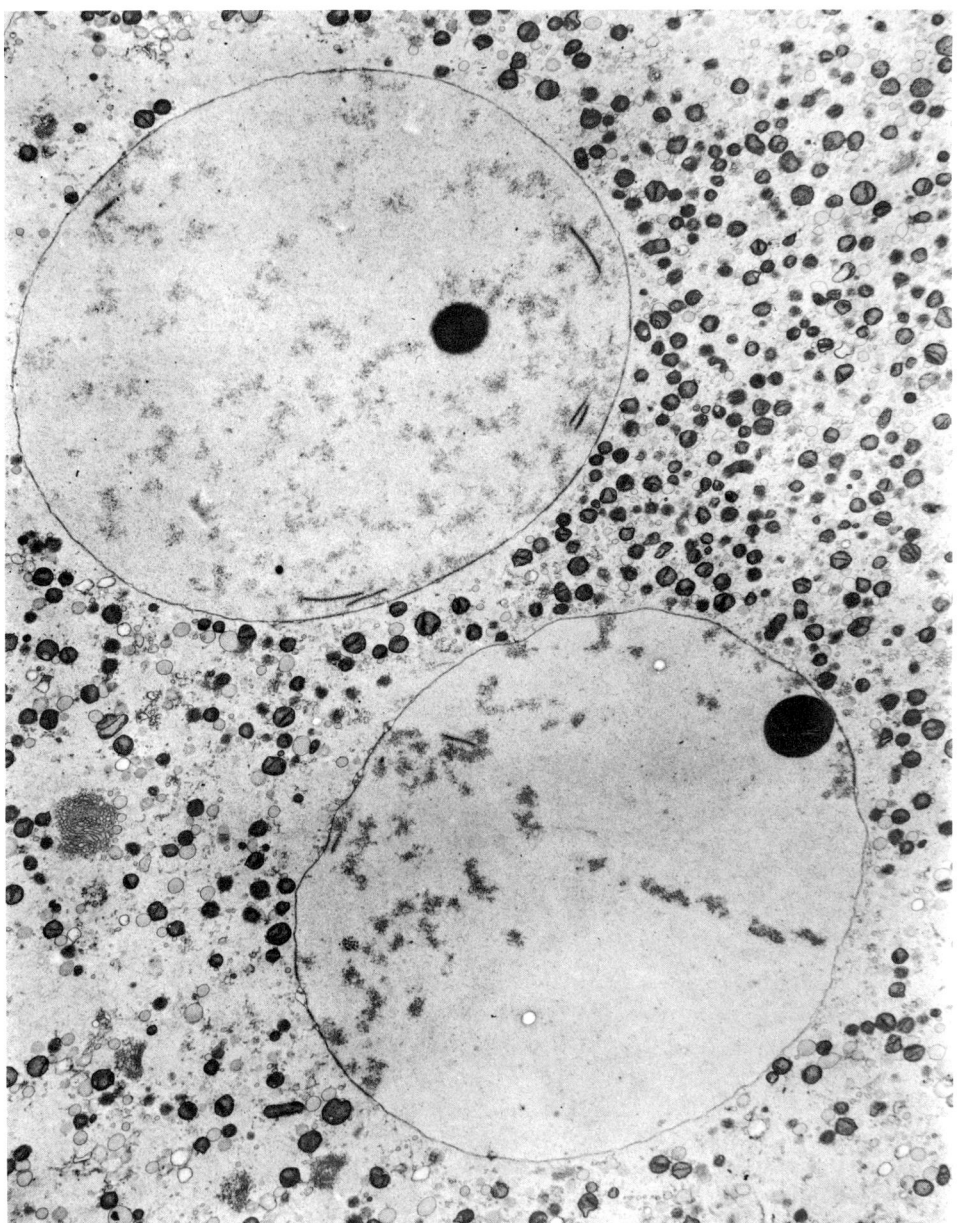

Fig. 3. Electron micrograph of the male and female pronuclei in a human ootid. The pronuclear material appears to be highly hydrated, although it is condensed in patches. A small black sphere, namely, the nucleolus, and some annulate lamellae are visible within each pronucleus. Numerous organelles are present in the cytoplasm adjacent to the pronuclei, and portions of a Golgi complex are visible near the lower left-hand corner of the photograph. × 5,400. Reproduced through the courtesy of Dr. Luciano Zamboni, University of California, Los Angeles, and the *Journal of Cell Biology*.

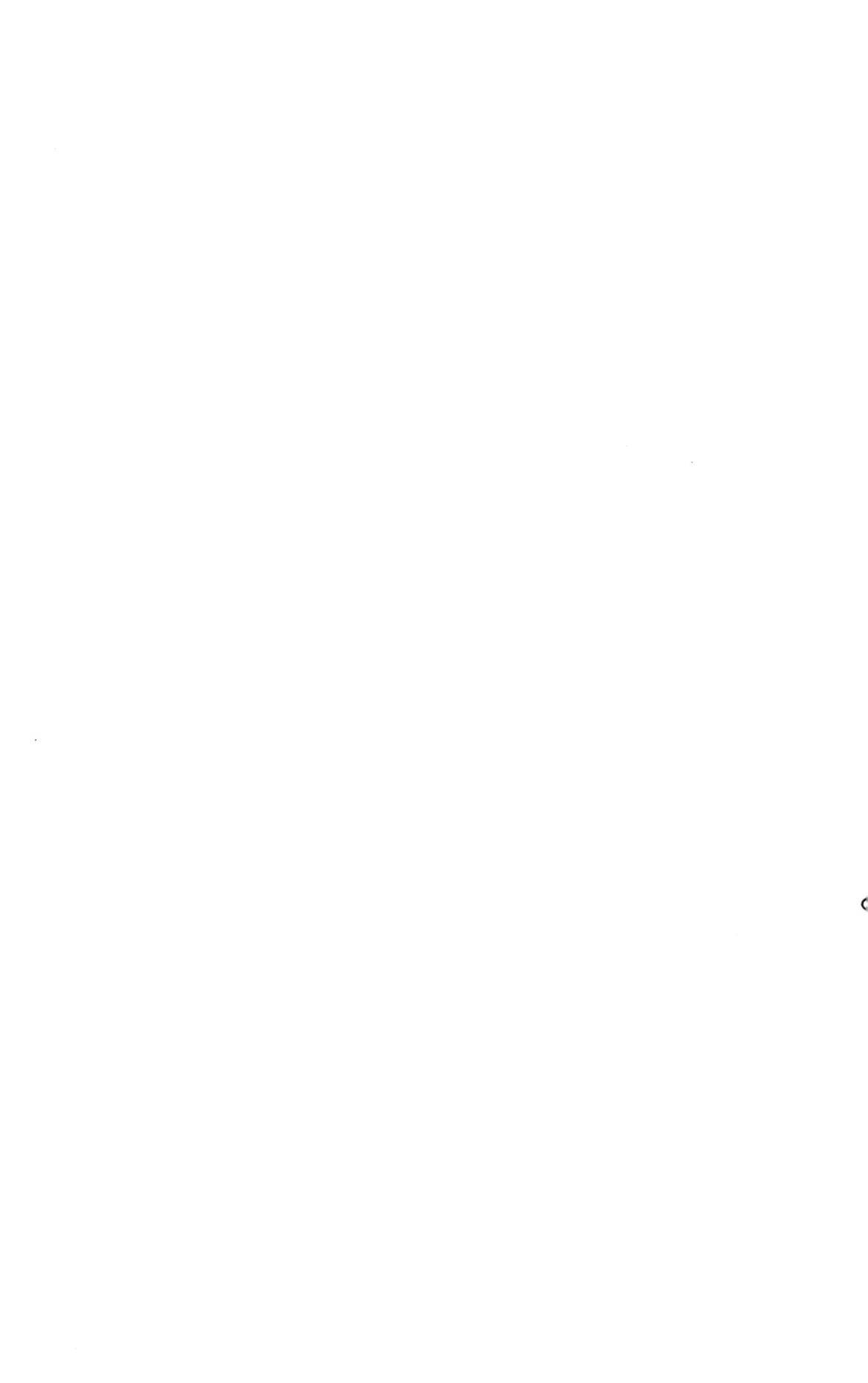

STAGE 2

Stage 2 comprises specimens from 2 cells up to the appearance of the segmentation cavity. Although no convenient designation is available for stage 2 specimens as a whole, two terms will be discussed briefly. The term "schizolig" (Gk., *schizo*, to cleave, and *oligos*, few) has been suggested to the writer by Professor William C. Korfmacher, St. Louis, to cover the earlier specimens. A schizolig may be defined as the developing organism in the early phases of cleavage, from 2 to about 11 cells. Presumably on the basis that at least a dozen surface elevations would be necessary to render a mulberry recognizable as such, the term "morula" (L. *morus*, mulberry) is not employed until at least 12 cells are present. (In the mouse, "embryos of 16 cells or more with no cavity are termed morulae;" Calarco and Brown, 1969.) In other words, the term "morula" is used for the organism from the more or less spherical, solid mass of a dozen or more cells up to the initial appearance of a segmentation cavity. Although the term "morula" is commonly used in mammalian embryology, Professor Blechschmidt, Göttingen, has pointed out to the writer that, because the amphibian morula gives rise to embryonic tissues only, the term is not appropriate in the case of mammals, in which non-embryonic structures (such as the chorion and the amnion) are also derived from the initial mass of cells. Professor Torrey agrees with this viewpoint, and it is proposed to avoid the term "morula" in the present work.

The diameter of stage 2 specimens before fixation is of the order of 175 micrometers; after fixation, it is approximately 120 (Hertig *et al.*, 1954). Indeed, shrinkage of as much as 50 per cent may occur in some instances (Menkin and Rock, 1948). Whether before or after fixation, the diameter at stage 2 may be expected to lie between 75 and 200 micrometers.

The volume of the protoplasmic mass (in the hamster) diminishes during cleavage, "from the time of ovulation until the blastocyst is formed" (Hamilton and Samuel, 1956). A similar statement, at least up to and including the schizolig, may be made in the case of the human (Table 5).

The organism proceeds along the uterine tube by means not entirely understood (and reviewed by Adams, 1960). It leaves the tube and enters the uterine cavity during the third or fourth day after ovulation, when the endometrium is early in the secretory phase (corresponding to the luteal phase of the ovarian cycle).

It has been shown experimentally (in the mouse, rat, and rabbit) that a blastomere isolated from the mammalian two-cell organism is capable of forming a complete embryo (Mulnard, 1965). Separation of the early blastomeres is believed to account for about one-third of all cases of monozygotic twinning in the human (Corner, 1955). Such twins should be dichorial and diamniotic (fig. 10). The fact that nearly 60 per cent of dichorial twins (whether monozygotic or dizygotic) have two unfused placentae "indicates that the zona pellucida . . . must have disappeared sufficiently long before implantation to allow the twins to become implanted in independent positions in the uterus" (Bulmer, 1970). Dizygotic twins, it may be mentioned, are believed to arise from two oocytes, from

TABLE 5. Total Protoplasmic Volume before and during the First Two Stages

Author and Specimen	Number of Cells	Diameter of Cell (μm)			Calculated volume (μm³) of each cell ($\frac{1}{6}\pi D^3$)	Total Protoplasmic Volume (μm³) ($\frac{1}{6}\pi D^3$)		
		Unfixed	Fixed	Sectioned		Unfixed	Fixed	Sectioned
Allen et al., 1930b: oocyte	1	102				554,500		
Hamilton, 1946: ootid	1	100				523,600		
Dickmann et al., 1965: ootid	1	108×90*				508,000		
Hertig et al., 1954: No. 8698	2	71	74 × 64	68 × 62	187,500 × 2	375,000	336,483	256,950
			80 × 56	70 × 50	171,833			
					164,650			
					143,800			
					113,150			
Khvatov, 1968	8		32		17,150 × 8		137,200	
Hertig et al., 1954: No. 8904	12	19.2			2,943 × 1	328,906		
		38.4			29,633 × 11			

*Estimated from photomicrograph.

a binucleate oocyte, or from a second polar body (Gedda, 1961).

As a result of ultrastructural and autoradiographic studies of cleavage in the mouse, it has been found that the nucleoli change in number, morphology, and activity during development (Hillman and Tasca, 1969). Multiple, fibrillary primary nucleoli are present in the early 2-cell embryo. The reticulated nucleoli of late 2-cell and of 4-cell embryos "can be considered, on the basis of their fine structure, to be definitive nucleoli" (*ibid.*).

The successive cleavage divisions do not occur synchronously, so that, in the pig, for example, specimens of 1, 2, 3, 4, 5, 6, 7, and 8 cells have been seen (Heuser and Streeter, 1929). The more precociously dividing cells appear to be those that give rise to the trophoblast (*ibid.*). Moreover, differences in the size of the blastomeres are observed.

There is reason to believe, however, that the blastomeres do not become determined very early in development. For example, it has been shown experimentally in the mouse (by cultivation *in vitro* of isolated blastomeres) that the ability to develop into trophoblastic cells is inherent in all blastomeres of the 4-cell and 8-cell organism. In other words, up to 8 cells, none of the blastomeres is yet determined to give rise to cells of the inner mass. It may be that the primary factor responsible for the determination of one of the two alternative routes of differentiation (trophoblast or inner cell mass) is simply the position (peripheral or internal) that a given cell occupies in the "morula" (Tarkowski, 1965a). Moreover, it has been possible in the mouse to unite two 16-cell organisms and obtain from them one giant, but otherwise perfectly normal, blastocyst (Tarkowski, 1965b). Fusion of mouse organisms "with close to 32 cells each" has also resulted in a single blastocyst (Mintz, 1964).

Cinematographic studies of the developing mouse have shown that embryos of about 8 cells become globular when certain cells tend to spread on the surface of the others (Mulnard, 1967). This indicates the beginning of a clear-cut distinction between two types of blastomeres, the central (which form the inner cell mass) and the peripheral (which constitute the trophoblast). In a baboon of approximately 32 cells (although classified as stage 2), large peripheral cells were identified as trophoblastic (Hendrickx and Kraemer, 1968).

In the human, the most significant specimens of stage 2 contain 2 and 12 cells respectively (Hertig et al., 1954).

The 2-cell specimen (No. 8698) was spherical and surrounded by a transparent zona pellucida (fig. 4). Two polar bodies were present. Each blastomere was nearly spherical. It has been maintained that the larger blastomere would probably divide first and hence may perhaps be trophoblastic (Hertig, 1968).

The 12-cell specimen (No. 8904) was perfectly spherical and surrounded by a clear zona pellucida. One blastomere, central in position and larger than the others, was presumed to be embryogenic, whereas the smaller cells were thought to be trophoblastic.

A number of human specimens of stage 2 found in atretic ovarian follicles were considered to be parthenogenetic by their authors (Häggström, 1922; Krafka, 1939; Herranz and Vázquez, 1964; Khvatov, 1968). Such a claim, however, has been disputed (Ashley, 1959), and it has been pointed out that polysegmentation, that is, cleavage-like conditions described as "pseudoparthenogenesis," are not infrequently encountered in moribund oocytes (Kampmeier, 1929). It is possible also that some instances of cleavage obtained *in vitro* may be pseudoparthenogenetic rather than due to actual fertilization by spermatozoa.

The presence of a Y chromosome in a "spread from a replicating blastomere" (Jacobson, Sites, and Arias-Bernal, 1970) has been claimed "but not convincingly demonstrated" (Brackett et al., 1972).

Several embryos of the baboon *(Papio sp.)* at stage 2 have been recorded (Hendrickx and Kraemer, 1968). They were obtained from either the uterine tubes or the uterine cavity, and they ranged from 4 to about 32 cells and from 140 to 202 micrometers in diameter.

Specimens of Stage 2 in Carnegie Collection

Carnegie specimens of stage 2, listed in the order of their serial numbers, are summarized in Table 6. Because of the great rarity of early specimens, abnormal embryos have been included but have been indicated as such. Double embedding in celloidin (C) and paraffin (P) was employed. The donors of Carnegie embryos have played an essential part in the work, and, in this as well as in subsequent tables, their names are included as an expression of gratitude for their cooperation.

Specimens of Stage 2 Already Described
(listed in order of numbers of cells present)

Specimens believed by their authors to have been parthenogenetic are indicated here by an asterisk.

2 cells, Carnegie No. 8260. Described by Menkin and Rock (1948). Produced by spermatozoal exposure of an oocyte *in vitro*. Diameter, 153 × 155 micrometers; vitellus, 100 × 113 (50 × 75 after fixation); thickness of zona pellucida, 23 (8 after fixation); blastomeres, 88 × 58 and 105 × 58 (63 × 39 and 66 × 36 after fixation); polar body, 18 × 10 after fixation. Another and similar specimen was lost before sectioning.

2 cells, Carnegie No. 8698 (fig. 4). Described by Hertig et al. (1954). Tubal. Diameter, 178.5 micrometers (122 × 88 after fixation; 111.6 × 75 after sectioning); blastomeres, 71 (74 × 64 and 80 × 56 after fixation; 68.3 × 61.6 and 70 × 50 after sectioning); polar bodies, 20 × 18 after fixation. A few cells of the corona radiata were present. Thick zona pellucida (18 micrometers in thickness before fixation). No spermatozoa were seen in the zona, and the possibility of parthenogenetic cleavage "cannot be entirely ruled out" (Dickmann et al., 1965). Two polar bodies. Whether the larger blastomere "is the one of trophoblastic potential is unknown but it is probable" (Hertig, 1968). Believed to be about 1½ days old.

2 cells. Illustrated by Shettles (1958 and 1960). Produced by seminal exposure of an oocyte *in vitro*.

2 cells undergoing cytolysis were produced parthenogenetically by Edwards et al. (1966)* from an oocyte cultured *in vitro*.

2 cells and 4 cells. Described by Häggström (1922),* who found them in atretic ovarian follicles of a 22-year-old woman.

3 cells, Carnegie No. 8500.1. Described by Menkin and Rock (1948). Produced by spermatozoal exposure of an oocyte *in vitro*. Diameter, 170 × 183 micrometers; vitellus, 103 × 127 (50 × 86 after fixation); thickness of zona pel-

TABLE 6. List of Specimens of Stage 2 in Carnegie Collection

Serial No.	Normality	Number of Blastomeres	Size of Fixed Specimen (micrometers)	Fixative	Cutting Medium	Thinness (micrometers)	Stain	Date and Donor	Reference
8190	abnormal	9	160 × 104	Alc. & Bouin	C-P	6	Iron h. or. G	1943, A.T. Hertig, Boston, Mass.	Hertig et al., 1954
8260	in vitro	2	50 × 75	Bouin	C-P	8	H.-E.	1944, J. Rock, Brookline, Mass.	Menkin & Rock, 1948
8450	abnormal	8	100 × 96	Alc. & Bouin	C-P	6	H.-E. phlox.	1947, A.T. Hertig, Boston, Mass.	Hertig et al., 1954
8452	abnormal	12	110 × 93	Alc. & Bouin	C-P	6	H.-E. phlox.	1946, A.T. Hertig, Boston, Mass.	Hertig et al., 1954
8500.1	in vitro	3	50 × 86	Bouin	C-P	8	H.-E.	1947, J. Rock, Brookline, Mass.	Menkin & Rock, 1948
8630	abnormal	5	104 × 94	Alc. & Bouin	C-P	6	H.-E.	1948, A.T. Hertig, Boston, Mass.	Hertig et al., 1954
8698	normal	2	122 × 88	Alc. & Bouin	C-P	6	H.-E.	1949, A.T. Hertig, Boston, Mass.	Hertig et al., 1954
8904	normal	12	115	Bouin	Specimen lost			1951, A.T. Hertig, Boston, Mass.	Hertig et al., 1954

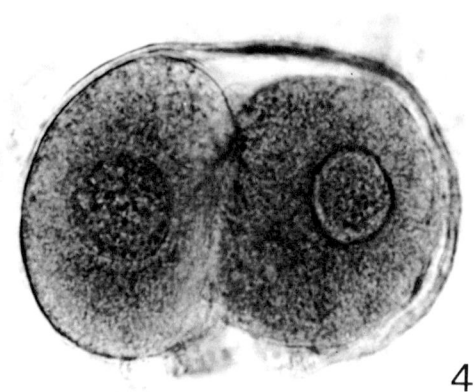
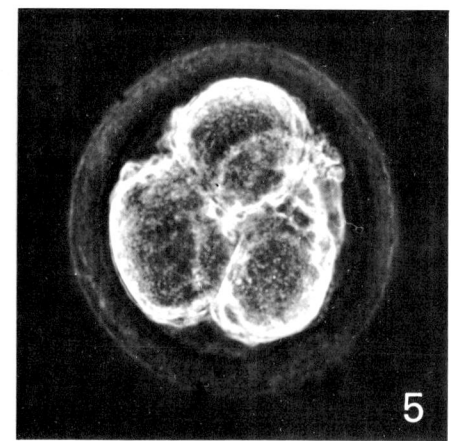

Fig. 4. Intact 2-cell schizolig showing zona pellucida and two polar bodies, the larger of which is clearly visible at the lower end of the cleavage line. No. 8698.

Fig. 5. Intact 4-cell schizolig. The granular zona pellucida can be distinguished. By courtesy of Dr. J. Lippes (Doyle et al., 1966) and the American Journal of Obstetrics and Gynecology.

lucida, 21; blastomeres, 97×73, 62×62, and 50×63 (66×49, 35×38, and 33×34 after fixation); a possible polar body, 14×9 after fixation. Another and similar specimen rapidly underwent degenerative changes.

3 cells. After seminal exposure of oocytes, Petrov (1968) found spermatozoal penetration of the zona pellucida after 2 hours, polyspermy in all cases, the first cleavage furrow after 20 hours, and three blastomeres after 26 hours.

4 cells. Illustrated by Krafka (1939),* who found it (within a zona pellucida) in an atretic ovarian follicle of a 7-year-old child.

4 cells. Described by Herranz and Vázquez (1964),* who found it (within a zona pellucida) in an atretic ovarian follicle of a 20-year-old woman.

4 cells. Illustrated by Way and Dawson (1959). Found in a routine vaginal smear. Well-marked zona pellucida.

4 cells. Illustrated by Shettles (1969). Produced by seminal exposure of an oocyte *in vitro*.

4 cells. Illustrated by Doyle et al. (1966). Found in middle third of uterine tube. Devoid of corona radiata. Granular zona pellucida (fig. 5).

5 to 12 cells. Pathological specimens of 5 (No. 8630), 8 (No. 8450), 9 (No. 8190), and 11 or 12 (No. 8452) cells have been featured by Hertig et al. (1954).

6 cells. Illustrated by Brackett et al. (1972). Produced by spermatozoal exposure of a follicular oocyte *in vitro*. Other specimens consisted of 2 to 12 cells and "a questionable morula undergoing degeneration."

8 cells. Noted by Khvatov (1968)* in an atretic ovarian follicle. Diameter (after fixation), 110×95 micrometers.

8 cells. Spermatozoal exposure of oocytes cultured *in vitro* resulted in specimens of 8 cells and also in some "early morulae and blastocysts" (Edwards and Fowler, 1970).

12 cells, Carnegie No. 8904. Described by Hertig *et al.* (1954). Uterine. Diameter, 172.8 micrometers (115.2 after fixation); blastomeres, 38.4 × 19.2. Clear zona pellucida (10 micrometers in thickness before fixation). Polar bodies not identified. No evidence of a segmentation cavity. A large, central blastomere was thought to be embryogenic, the other cells trophoblastic. Specimen lost during preparation. Believed to be about 3 days old.

16 cells. Specimens ranging from 1 to "16 or more" cells were produced by spermatozoal exposure of pre-ovulatory oocytes *in vitro* (Edwards, Steptoe, and Purdy, 1970). Photographs of a 4- and an 8-cell specimen were included.

STAGE 3

Stage 3 consists of the free (that is, unattached) blastocyst, a term employed as soon as the segmentation cavity appears. The blastocyst, then, is the hollow mass of cells from the initial appearance of the segmentation cavity (stage 3) to just before the completion of implantation (at a subsequent stage). The segmentation cavity begins by the coalescence of intercellular spaces when the organism has acquired about 32 cells. In *in vitro* studies, a cavity formed in some human embryos at 16–20 cells (Edwards, 1972).

It is important to realize that the cavity of the mammalian blastocyst is not the counterpart of the amphibian or the avian blastocoel. In the bird, the blastocoel is the limited space between the epiblast and the primary endoderm (Pasteels, 1945). The cavity of the mammalian blastocyst, however, corresponds to the subgerminal space together with the area occupied by the yolk (Torrey, personal communication, 1972).

The mammalian blastocyst differs from a blastula in that its cells have already differentiated into at least two types (trophoblastic and embryonic cells proper). Moreover, "all Eutherian mammals are fundamentally alike in their manner of cleavage and blastocyst formation and even the Marsupialia follow practically the same course" (Mossman, 1937).

During stage 3 the trophoblastic cells, owing to their peripheral position, are distinguishable from the embryonic cells proper. The latter become surrounded by the trophoblastic cells and lie within an inner mass. Studies of various mammals have indicated that the inner cell mass represents more than the embryo itself, insofar as it constitutes "a germinal mass of various potentialities" that continues for a time to add cells to the more precociously developed trophoblast (Heuser and Streeter, 1929 and 1941). The inner cell mass gives origin to the primary endoderm, and its remainder (the "formative cells") constitutes the epiblast. The epiblastic cells soon become aligned into what is frequently described as the "germ disc." These various relationships are summarized in figure 24. Duplication of the inner cell mass probably accounts for most instances of monozygotic twinning (Corner, 1955; Bulmer, 1970). Such twins should be monochorial but diamniotic (fig. 10).

Heuser and Streeter (1941) emphasized an important point by using stage 3 as an example: "The blastocyst form is not to be thought of solely in terms of the next succeeding stage in development. It is to be remembered that at all stages the embryo is a living organism, that is, it is a going concern with adequate mechanisms for its maintenance as of that time." It is no less true, however, that changes occur "in the growing organism and its environment which provide critically for the future survival of the organism" (Reynolds, 1954). Indeed, such morphological and functional changes during development "critically anticipate future morphological and functional requirements for the survival and welfare of the organism" (*ibid.*).

It is believed that, in the mouse, the blastomeres attain the ability to secrete the blastocystic fluid after a definite number of cleavages, namely, at the end of the fifth and at the beginning of the sixth mitotic cycle (Tarkowski, 1965a).

By cinematographic analysis of the developing mouse, it has been shown that, when the organism consists of about 32 cells, small cavities unite to form the beginning of the segmentation cavity (Mulnard, 1967). In other words, the solid phase of development (in the mouse) "ends at about 28 to 32 cells, when fluid begins to accumulate beneath the trophoblast cells" (Lewis and Wright, 1935). As the blastocyst develops, it undergoes expansions and contractions. When contracted, a "pseudomorula" of about 100 cells may be seen (Mulnard, 1967).

Hill and Tribe (1924) found that the so-called morula of the cat showed no appreciable increase in size during the formation of the blastocyst cavity, nor were the cells of the embryonic knot more compactly arranged after than before the appearance of that cavity. They concluded that "no mere flowing together of inter- or intra-cellular spaces or vacuoles is a sufficient explanation of its origin in Felis" and that an additional factor, namely, cytolysis of certain of the central cells, is also involved.

It has been suggested that, in the mouse, the contents of the blastocyst cavity "are derived from cytoplasmic vesicles which increase in number subsequent to fertilization and then decrease in number as they coalesce and release their contents into intercellular spaces" (Calarco and Brown, 1969).

It has been found by electron microscopy of the developing rat that the "blastocyst cavity first appears as small irregularly shaped cavities occurring between two or three cells. There may be one or two of these cavities initially. The cells encompassing the cavities have pronounced junctional complexes at their juxtazonal borders" (Schlafke and Enders, 1967). The formation of junctional complexes, which is regarded as the first sign of blastocyst formation, is found very early in the rat, when the embryo consists of only eight cells, although the first indication of a cavity, as opposed to intercellular spaces, is not seen until after another series of cell divisions.

Moreover, these ultrastructural studies of the developing rat have emphasized a continual change in cytology. However, "the cytological changes reflect the total differentiation of the fertilized ovum into blastocyst cytoplasm to a much more striking extent than they do differentiation of any particular cell type." In other words, "no [cytological] evidence for predetermined regions of the cytoplasm of the ovum was obtained" (Schlafke and Enders, 1967).

In the pig embryo it has been shown that, in general, "during the first seven days the cells undergo about eight divisions, that is, they divide about once a day" (Heuser and Streeter, 1929). A similar generalization may be made for the human embryo during stages 1 to 3, and also for the baboon (Hendrickx, 1971). In the case of the baboon, "there is a close correlation between age and cell number," although "there is no consistent relationship between age and size for these stages of development" (*ibid.*). Although "mouse embryos developing *in vivo* from the 2-cell to the blastocyst stage showed a constant cell doubling time of about 10 h.," embryos cultured *in vitro* over the same period slowed to a doubling time of about 24 hours (Bowman and McLaren, 1970). Actually, however, the *in vivo* graph (their fig. 1), which extended up to 64 cells only, is very similar to that shown here for the human (fig. 6), and further data would be required to find out whether the mouse

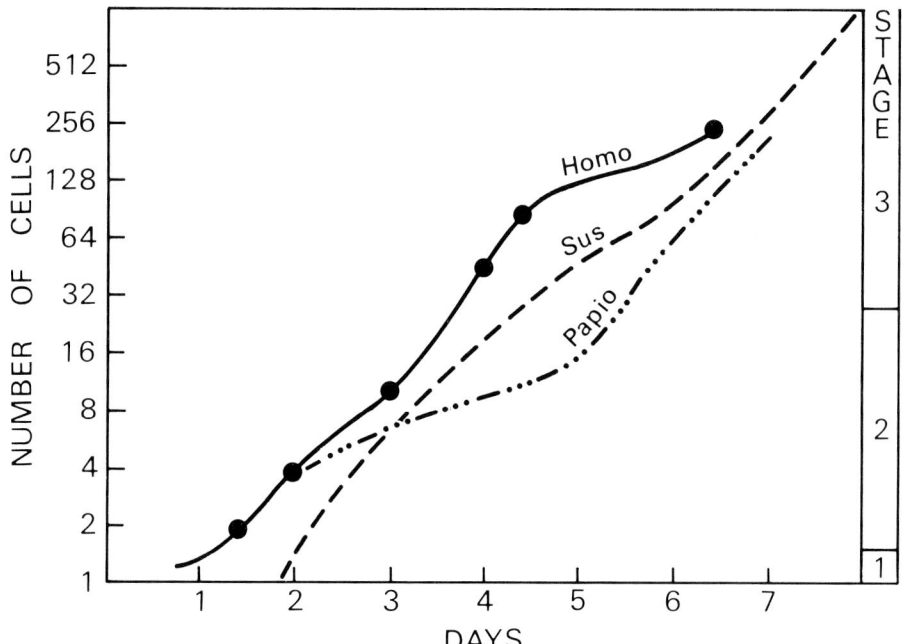

Fig. 6. Graph showing presumed age plotted against number of cells. The continuous line is based on six human embryos: 8698, Doyle et al., 8904, 8794, 8663, and Krafka. The interrupted lines indicate pig (Streeter, 1929) and baboon (Hendrickx, 1971) embryos. In each case the rate of cleavage during the first week is not much faster than one division per day.

embryo really undergoes division at a more rapid rate.

Although too few specimens are available to make practicable a precise study of increase in size of the human blastocyst during development, such an increase has been demonstrated in the case of the mouse (Dickson, 1966). In the human, all that can be stated at present is that an increase occurs in maximum diameter from 100–200 micrometers at stages 2 and 3 to 300–450 micrometers at stage 5a.

In stage 3, the zona pellucida may be either present or absent. In the baboon, the zona is shed late in stage 3 (day 7 or 8) "in contrast to estimated day 5 in man" (Hendrickx, 1971).

In the human, the most significant specimens of stage 3 are a 58-cell and a 107-cell blastocyst (Hertig et al., 1954).

In the 58-cell specimen (No. 8794), 53 of the cells were trophoblastic whereas five were embryonic. The latter comprised the inner cell mass, which was located eccentrically within the segmentation cavity but had not yet assumed a truly polar position.

In the 107-cell specimen (No. 8663), 99 of the cells were trophoblastic, and, of these, 69 were mural in position and 30 were polar, that is, covering the embryonic pole. Eight of the 107 cells were embryonic, and were characterized by their larger size and by the presence of intracytoplasmic vacuoles. Moreover, the eight cells comprised three types: "obvious primitive, vacuolated ectoderm [epiblast]; flattened primitive endoderm; and a large indifferent cell, presumably a [primordial] germ cell" (Hertig, 1968). In addition, of the 30 polar trophoblastic cells, four which are situated "ventral and lateral to the formative cells ... may actually be of primitive endodermal type" (Hertig et al., 1954).

A comparison of stage 3 embryos with those of stage 5 makes it clear that the surface of the inner cell mass that is adjacent to the polar trophoblast represents the dorsal surface of the embryo, and the surface of the mass that faces the segmentation cavity represents the ventral surface. In other words, "dorsalization," or "dorsoventrality," becomes apparent during stage 3 (O'Rahilly, 1970). The possibility should be kept in mind, however, that the inner cell mass can travel around the inside of the trophoblastic layer (Kirby, Potts, and Wilson, 1967).[1]

Sex chromatin has been "tentatively identified" in two *in vitro* human blastocysts (Edwards, 1972).

Five embryos of the baboon *(Papio sp.)* at stage 3 have been described (Hendrickx and Kraemer, 1968). They ranged from 126 to 160 micrometers in length and from 96 to 144 micrometers in width. "The length of this stage [days 5 to 8] is approximately 3 days longer in the baboon than has been estimated for man" (Hendrickx, 1971).

Since the above chapter was written, the results of a symposium on the biology of the blastocyst have been published (Blandau, 1971).

SPECIMENS OF STAGE 3 IN CARNEGIE COLLECTION

Certain data concerning the Carnegie specimens of stage 3 are summarized in Table 7.

[1] "Alice remained looking thoughtfully at the mushroom for a minute, trying to make out which were the two sides of it; and, as it was perfectly round, she found this a very difficult question" (Lewis Carroll: *Alice's Adventures in Wonderland*).

SPECIMENS OF STAGE 3 ALREADY DESCRIBED

(listed in order of numbers of cells present)

Ca. 32 cells. Described by Shettles (1956 and 1960). Produced by seminal exposure of an oocyte *in vitro*. Zona pellucida denuded of corona and cumulus cells. "Early segmentation cavity."

Ca. 50 cells. Described by Shettles (1957) as due to "parthenogenetic cleavage." Zona pellucida denuded of corona and cumulus cells. Diameter, including zona, 150 micrometers. "Early segmentation cavity."

58 cells, Carnegie No. 8794. Described by Hertig *et al.* (1954). Uterine. Diameter, 230 × 190 micrometers (108 × 86 after fixation; 101 × 73.3 after sectioning); diameters of blastomeres varied from 15 to 23 after sectioning; polar bodies, 18 after fixation. Zona pellucida intact while fresh but partly deficient after fixation (fig. 7). Two polar bodies. Early segmentation cavity. Believed to be about 4 days old.

100 cells. Described by Khvatov (1967). Tubal. Diameter, 126 × 100 × 70 micrometers. Nuclei in trophoblastic blastomeres darker (with hematoxylin and eosin). Said to be female, "based on current studies concerning sex chromatin."

"More than 100 cells." Two such blastocysts were produced by spermatozoal exposure of oocytes cultured *in vitro*, and "bodies resembling sex chromatin were seen in a few nuclei" (Steptoe, Edwards, and Purdy, 1971; Edwards, 1972).

107 cells, Carnegie No. 8663. Described by Hertig *et al.* (1954). Uterine. No zona pellucida (fig. 8). Diameter, 153 × 115 micrometers (103 × 80 after fixation;

TABLE 7. List of Specimens of Stage 3 in Carnegie Collection

Serial No.	Normality	Number of Blastomeres	Size of Fixed Specimen (micrometers)	Fixative	Cutting Medium	Thinness (micrometers)	Stain	Date and Donor	Reference
8663	normal	107	103 × 80	Alc. & Bouin	C-P	6	H.-E.	1949, A.T. Hertig, Boston, Mass.	Hertig et al., 1954
8794	normal	58	108 × 86	Alc. & Bouin	C-P	6	H.-E.	1950, A.T. Hertig, Boston, Mass.	Hertig et al., 1954

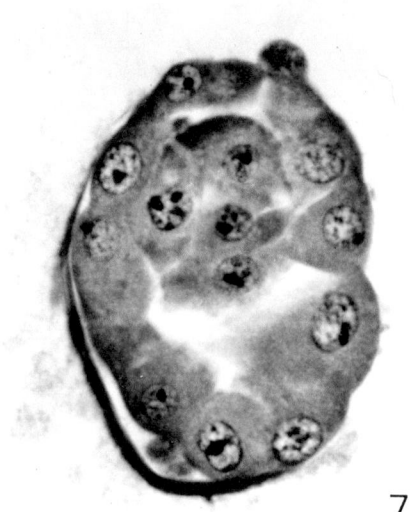 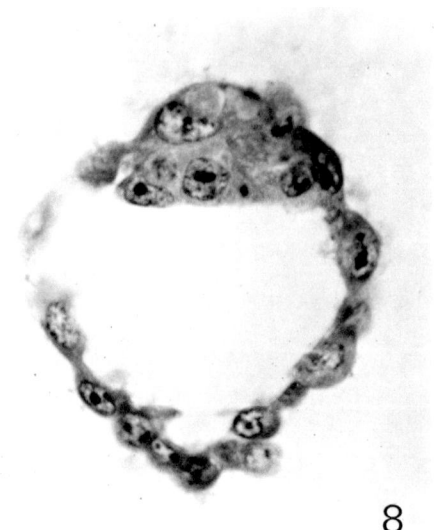

Fig. 7. Section through a 58-cell blastocyst (No. 8794). The zona pellucida is visible on the lower left-hand part of the mass, where a polar body can also be recognized. The inner cell mass can be seen above the segmentation cavity. The more peripherally situated cells are trophoblastic.

Fig. 8. Section through a 107-cell blastocyst (No. 8663). The zona pellucida is no longer present. The segmentation cavity is now quite large. The embryonic pole, characterized by the inner cell mass, is shown uppermost. The peripheral layer of cells constitutes the trophoblast.

91.6 × 83.3 after sectioning); diameters of blastomeres varied from 8 to 21. Large segmentation cavity (58 micrometers). Embryonic mass composed of 8 cells: epiblastic (ectodermal), endodermal, and a presumed primordial germ cell (Hertig, 1968). Believed to be about 4½ days old. Khvatov (1967), without further elaboration, claimed: "according to photographs, should be of the male sex." Smith (1970, fig. 15), without further justification, claimed that a cytoplasmic vacuole was "the first indication toward an amniotic space."

Ca. 200 to 300 cells. Described briefly by Krafka (1942). Tubal. Diameter, 120 × 180 micrometers. Zona pellucida intact. Some adherent granulosa cells. Described as "solid" but the large number of cells suggests that it should have had a segmentation cavity (it may be a "pseudomorula," i.e., a contracted blastocyst); hence it is included here in stage 3.

STAGE 4

Although the criteria for the first three stages are those of the first three horizons, it has not proved practicable in stages 4 to 10 to retain the criteria for horizons IV to X. It may be pointed out that this abandonment had already been begun by Hertig, Rock, and Adams (1956) and by Heuser and Corner (1957).

Stage 4, the onset of implantation, is reserved for the attaching blastocyst, which is probably 5½ to 6 days old.

It should be noted at the outset that certain specimens that are now listed in stages 5a and 5b (Hertig, Rock, and Adams, 1956) were formerly included in Horizon IV. In other words, because such specimens represent "significantly different stages of development" (*ibid.*), they have been transferred, and, as a result, stage 4 has been made more restricted. Healing of the uterine epithelium over the conceptus, for example, is too variable and has been eliminated as a criterion for stage 5; it usually occurs after horizon VI has begun (Böving, 1965).

Implantation is a highly complicated and ill-understood phenomenon "by which the conceptus is transported to its site of attachment, held there, oriented properly, and then attached by adhesion, trophoblastic penetration, spread, proliferation, envelopment of vessels, and other developments of the placenta, both conceptal and maternal parts" (Böving, 1963). In this broad sense, implantation includes at least stages 4 and 5.

Implantation, then, includes (a) dissolution of the zona pellucida, and contact and attachment (adhesion) between the blastocyst and the endometrium; (b) penetration; and (c) migration of the blastocyst through the endometrium. On the basis of comparative studies, it has been suggested (Böving, 1965) that stage 4 might be subdivided into these three phases. Human (but not macaque) implantation is interstitial in type, that is, the blastocyst comes to lie entirely within the substance of the endometrium. In the human (as also in the macaque), implantation occurs into an edematous, nondeciduous endometrium. In other words, decidualization takes place at the end of implantation.

In his important study of the early development of the Primates, Hill (1932) concluded as follows:

"The outstanding feature of the early human blastocyst is its extraordinary precocity as exemplified . . . in the relations it very early acquires to the uterine lining and in the remarkably early differentiation of its trophoblast and its extra-embryonal mesoderm. It is no longer content to undergo its development in the uterine lumen as does that of all the lower Primates, but, whilst still quite minute, burrows its way through the uterine epithelium and implants itself in the very vascular subepithelial decidual tissue of the uterus. Therein it forms for itself a decidual cavity and undergoes its subsequent development, completely embedded in the maternal tissue. In this way the Primate germ reaches the acme of its endeavour to maintain itself in the uterus and to obtain an adequate supply of nutriment at the earliest possible moment."

The mammalian stage 2 organism and the early blastocyst are surrounded by an intact zona pellucida, which disappears at the beginning of implantation. Hence, implantation "is taken as beginning when the zona pellucida is lost and the trophoblast is in contact with the uterine epithelium throughout its circumference" (Young, Whicher, and Potts, 1968). Although claims have been made that the blastocyst emerges from its zona pellucida by "shedding" or by "hatching," it has more recently been maintained that, at least in the case of the mouse, the zona undergoes rapid dissolution all around the blastocyst (Reinius, 1967) *in situ*, that is, at the actual site of implantation (Potts and Wilson, 1967).

In the mouse, after the blastocyst becomes attached at random to the uterine epithelium, it is believed that the inner cell mass can travel around the inside of the trophoblastic shell (presumably somewhat like a satellite gear). Although "the nature of the stimulus responsible for the final orientation of the inner cell mass is unknown," it is postulated that the final position "is determined either by a morphogenetic gradient across the vertical axis of the uterus or by changes in the trophoblast associated with its attachment to the underlying tissues, or by both" (Kirby, Potts, and Wilson, 1967).

The implantation site has been studied by electron microscopy in several mammals, such as the mouse. The cell membranes of the trophoblast and uterine epithelium become intimately related, and large cytoplasmic inclusions are found in the trophoblastic cells. "The ultrastructural changes taking place at implantation suggest that there may be a high degree of permeability between maternal and embryonic cells. . . . In addition there may be an exchange of cellular material between uterus and embryo" (Potts, 1968).

After the zona pellucida has become dissolved, the surface membranes of the trophoblast and uterine epithelium are separated by a narrow interval (in the mouse). When the membranes "lie within 150 Å apart over wide areas, then the blastocyst attachment has occurred" (Reinius, 1967). This first morphological sign of implantation can be detected only by electron microscopy, however.

In at least some macaque specimens a distinction between cytotrophoblast and syncytiotrophoblast [1] can be made (Heuser and Streeter, 1941, e.g., No. C-520, their fig. 38). Moreover, amniogenic cells can be detected "separating from the trophoblast above and . . . distinct from the germ disk" (*ibid.*, No. C-610, their fig. 53). Finally, formative or epiblastic ("germ disc") cells and endoderm can be distinguished (*ibid.*, No. C-520, their fig. 40).

Of the several macaque specimens of stage 4 that have been described, in one instance (No. C-560), the uterine epithelium at the site of attachment showed a disturbed arrangement of its nuclei. Moreover, the cytoplasm had become paler, which was taken to indicate beginning cytolysis. In the conceptus, the site of attachment was formed by syncytiotrophoblast, which is initially formed by the coalescence of polar trophoblast (Hertig, 1968). Some of the increased number of nuclei appeared to

---

[1] "Syncytium is now properly used to designate the situation in which a multinucleate condition is established by the fusion of initially separate cells. Plasmodium, on the other hand, is the term applied to a mass of multinucleate protoplasm that has arisen as the result of repeated nuclear division without consequential partitioning of the associated cytoplasm" (Boyd and Hamilton, 1966). With regard to the origin of the syncytium in the human placenta, it has been pointed out that "being derived from the cells in the wall of the blastocyst, all the trophoblast was initially constituted by individual and separate cellular elements" (*ibid.*).

have been released from the uterine epithelium and then engulfed by the rapidly expanding trophoblast. Within the cavity of the blastocyst, disintegrating embryonic cells were interpreted as a mechanical accident due to displacement of the cells.

At the site of attachment, fused multinucleated cells of the uterine epithelium constitute a "symplasma," which fuses with the syncytiotrophoblast (in macaque No. C-610, and also in the rabbit; in the latter it has been studied by electron miscroscopy by Larsen, 1970).

A specimen of stage 4 in the baboon has been illustrated (Hendrickx, 1971). The single layer of abembryonic trophoblast was continuous with the cytotrophoblast dorsally. The syncytiotrophoblast was in contact with the uterine epithelium, which had lost its columnar appearance. Moreover, as much as one-half of the surface portion of the uterine cells had disappeared at the site of attachment. The inner cell mass showed occasional "endoblastic" cells bordering the blastocyst cavity. The age of the specimen was estimated as 9 days.

In the human, the only report of stage 4 seems to be two not altogether satisfactory photographs in a Supplement to *Ovum humanum* (Shettles, 1960, figs. 65 and 66). One illustration is captioned "attachment of the blastocyst to the uterine epithelium during the sixth day after ovulation. The encapsulating zona pellucida has disappeared." The second figure is a high-power view to show that "pseudopodia-like protoplasmic projections from blastocyst traverse the adjacent zona pellucida at area of contact with endometrium."

Clearly a need exists for the finding and recording of a good specimen of stage 4 in the human, comparable to those in the macaque illustrated by Heuser and Streeter (1941, Plate 3, fig. 31, and Plate 5, fig. 48).

STAGE 5

Stage 5 comprises embryos that are implanted to a varying degree but are previllous, i.e., that do not yet show chorionic villi. Such embryos are believed to be 7 to 12 days old. The chorion varies from about 0.3 to 1 mm, and the embryonic disc measures approximately 0.1 to 0.2 mm in diameter. The significant dimensions of Carnegie specimens of stage 5 are listed in Table 8. The external and internal diameters of the chorion are listed as "chorion" and "chorionic cavity," respectively. Additional features of stage 5 include the definite appearance of the amniotic cavity and the formation of extra-embryonic mesoblast. The appearances at stages 2 to 5 are shown in figure 9.

Implantation, which began in stage 4, is the characteristic feature of stage 5. It should be appreciated that both maternal and embryonic tissues are involved in the complex process of implantation: "in the normal process they are mutually supporting and neither can be regarded as chiefly responsible" (Boyd and Hamilton, 1970). An indication of a decidual reaction appears during stage 5 and, from this time onwards, the term "decidua" (used by William Hunter) is commonly employed. The decidua, at least in the human, "is a tissue made up of endometrial connective tissue cells which have enlarged and become rounded or polyhedral due to the accumulation of glycogen or lipoids within their cytoplasm, and which occur either in pregnancy, pseudo-pregnancy or in artificially or pathologically stimulated deciduomata" (Mossman, 1937).

Heuser's technique of opening the uterus laterally and searching for a young conceptus has been described on several occasions (e.g., by Hertig, Rock, and Adams, 1956, p. 438; and by Heard, 1957, p. 5).

No correlation has been found between the side of the uterus on which the conceptus becomes implanted and the ovary from which the oocyte originated (Hertig and Rock, 1949). Normal specimens, however, are more commonly found implanted on the posterior wall of the uterus, abnormal ones on the anterior wall (*ibid.*). Both walls are considered to be antimesometrial in comparison with a bicornuate uterus (Mossman, 1937). Furthermore, "it is interesting to note that cases are known of a double discoid placenta in man very similar to that of the monkey. It seems entirely possible that in some cases the human blastocyst may attach both dorsally and ventrally and therefore fail to undergo complete interstitial implantation" (*ibid.*).

The trophoblast from stages 4 and 5 onwards comprises two chief varieties, namely, cytotrophoblast and syncytiotrophoblast. That the latter is derived from the former had long been suspected and has more recently been shown by organ culture (Tao, 1962, cited by Hertig, 1968; Tao and Hertig, 1965) and also indicated by electron microscopy (Enders, 1965).

An amniotic cavity is found by stage 5. If duplication of the embryo occurs after the differentiation of the amnion, the resulting monozygotic twins should be monochorial and monoamniotic (fig. 10). It has been estimated that the frequency of monoamniotic twins among monozygotic twins is about four per cent (Bulmer, 1970). About once in every 400 monozygotic twin pregnancies, the duplication is incomplete and conjoined

TABLE 8. Significant Dimensions (in millimeters) of Carnegie Specimens of Stage 5

Stage	5a	5a	5a	5b	5b	5b	5b	5c	5c	5c	5c	5c
Serial No.	8225	8020	8155	8215	8171	8004	9350	7699	7950	7700	8558	8330
Age in days	7	7	8	9	9	9	9	11	12	12	12	12
Chorion	0.33 × 0.306 × 0.12	0.45 × 0.30 × 0.125	0.306 × 0.210 × 0.15	0.525 × 0.498 × 0.207	0.422 × 0.404 × 0.256	0.582 × 0.45 × 0.31	0.599 × 0.58 × 0.36	1.026 × 0.713 × 0.515	0.75 × 0.45	0.948 × 0.835 × 0.54	0.96 × 0.52	0.85 × 0.65
Chorionic cavity	0.228 × 0.20 × 0.03	0.288 × 0.186 × 0.044	0.168 × 0.082 × 0.066	0.228 × 0.21 × 0.10	0.164 × 0.138 × 0.08	0.312 × 0.185 × 0.12	0.3 × 0.1 × 0.1	0.48 × 0.336 × 0.276	0.40 × 0.26	0.55 × 0.498 × 0.425	0.58 × 0.36	0.46 × 0.40
Trophoblast	0.006 — 0.086	0.003 — 0.09	0.003 — 0.08	0.013 — 0.16	0.04 — 0.13	0.035 — 0.175		0.064 — 0.153	0.04 — 0.15	0.0125 — 0.185	0.02 — 0.28	0.10 — 0.24
Embryonic disc	0.09 × 0.078 × 0.036	0.126 × 0.092 × 0.044	0.09 × 0.05 × 0.03	0.084 × 0.052 × 0.05	0.114 × 0.088 × 0.046	0.132 × 0.10 × 0.046	0.132 × 0.09 × 0.05	0.138 × 0.138 × 0.089	0.16 × 0.07	0.204 × 0.165 × 0.045	0.22 × 0.08	0.216 × 0.063
Amniotic cavity	0.06 × 0.054 × 0.006	0.025 × 0.024 × 0.003	0.048 × 0.032 × 0.02	0.05 × 0.048 × 0.022	0.04 × 0.036 × 0.024	0.078 × 0.066 × 0.012		0.108 × 0.099 × 0.024	0.02 × 0.014	0.174 × 0.14 × 0.0125	0.216 × 0.036	0.16 × 0.05
Exocoelomic cavity				0.08 × 0.023	0.043 × 0.06	absent		0.246 × 0.168 × 0.124	0.33 × 0.19	0.474 × 0.41 × 0.29	0.49 × 0.30	0.35 × 0.31
Reference	Hertig and Rock (1945b)	Hertig and Rock (1945a)	Hertig and Rock (1949)	Hertig and Rock (1945c)	Hertig and Rock (1949)	Hertig and Rock (1945a)	Heuser (1956)	Hertig and Rock (1941)	Hertig, Rock, and Adams (1956)	Hertig and Rock (1941)	Hertig, Rock, and Adams (1956)	Hertig, Rock, and Adams (1956)

STAGE 5

("Siamese") twins (e.g., the second specimen of Shaw, 1932) result.

The following description of stage 5 is based largely on the work of Hertig and Rock, in whose publications (1941, 1945a, 1949) much additional information (including descriptions of the ovaries, uterine tubes, and uterus) may be found. Based on the condition of the trophoblast and its vascular relationships, stage 5 is subdivided into three groups: 5a, 5b, and 5c (Hertig, Rock, and Adams, 1956).

Although a brief description of the trophoblast at each stage is provided in this account, the main emphasis is devoted to the embryo itself. This is all the more justifiable in view of the circumstance that comprehensive books on the human trophoblast (Hertig, 1968) and the human placenta (Boyd and Hamilton, 1970) have recently been published.

STAGE 5a

The characteristic feature of subdivision 5a is that the trophoblast is still solid, in the sense that lacunae have not yet appeared. Specimens of this stage are believed to be 7 to 8 days old. The chorion is less than 0.5 mm in its greatest diameter, and the embryonic disc is approximately 0.1 mm in diameter. Because of the collapse of the conceptus during implantation, the blastocyst cavity is flattened.

The rarity of specimens of stage 5a has been attributed to the circumstance that they are "impossible to discern in the fresh, and probably often unrecognizable even after fixation" (Hertig, 1968).

Endometrium. The endometrial stroma is edematous (fig. 12). Two specimens (Nos. 8020 and 8225) show early, superficial implantation. The conceptus has eroded the surface epithelium of the uterus and has just penetrated the underlying stroma (fig. 13). Apparently an attempt has been made by the maternal epithelium to repair the defect, and occasional mitotic figures are found. A portion of the conceptus, however, is still exposed to the uterine cavity. A third specimen (No. 8155) shows later, interstitial implantation. The conceptus is almost embedded within the endometrium, so that its abembryonic pole, which is barely exposed, is nearly flush with the epithelial lining of the uterine cavity (fig. 14).

Trophoblast. The trophoblast may encroach on the surrounding endometrial glands. At the abembryonic pole, the wall of the conceptus is merely a thin layer of cells which resembles mesothelium. Because this region is not in contact with maternal tissue, it probably presents the structure of the wall of the blastocyst as it was at the time of implantation. Owing to the collapse of the blastocyst during implantation, the mesothelioid layer is closely applied to the ventral surface of the embryonic disc (fig. 13).

As the mesothelioid layer is traced laterally, it becomes continuous first with indifferent trophoblastic cells, which, at the embryonic pole, become differentiated into cytotrophoblast and syncytiotrophoblast. Definitive trophoblast is found only in the area of endometrial contact, presumably under the influence of an endometrial factor. A ventrodorsal gradient of trophoblastic differentiation is noticeable. In other words, the most highly developed trophoblast tends to be found deeply, i.e., away from the uterine cavity.

The cytotrophoblast is located nearer the embryonic disc. The cells are large and polyhedral, and show distinct cell boundaries. Mitotic figures are moderately frequent.

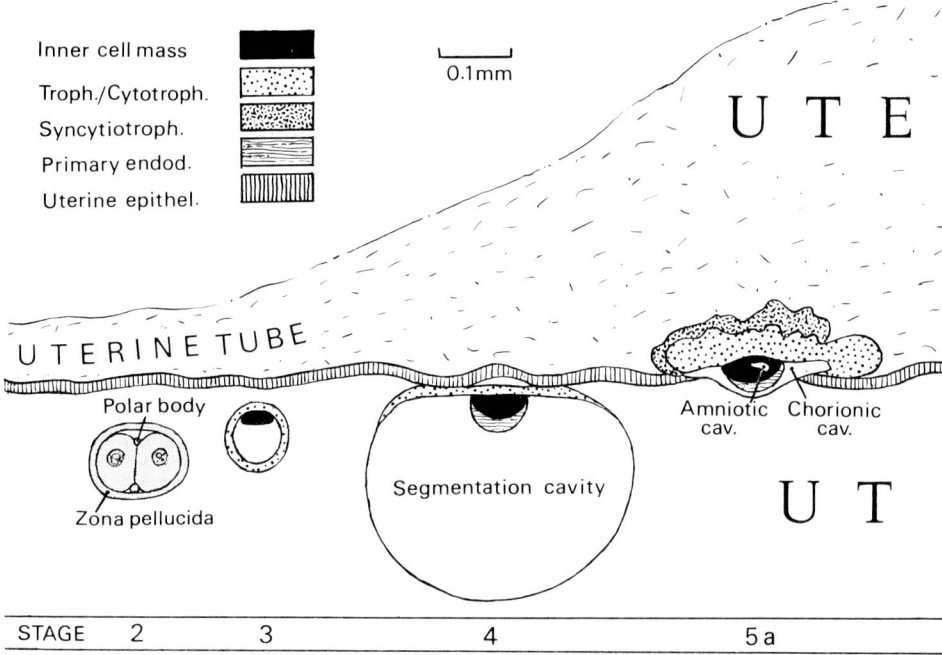

Fig. 9. Drawings of the embryo from stage 2 to stage 5c to show implantation. The drawings, which are all at the same scale of magnification, are based on human specimens, with the exception of stage 4, for which a macaque blastocyst has been used.

The syncytiotrophoblast is described by Hertig (1968) as "invasive, ingestive, and digestive." It presents a dark, homogeneous cytoplasm, and large, densely stained nuclei. No mitotic figures are seen. Near the maternal tissue, the syncytiotrophoblastic mass displays numerous small nuclei, which appear to be formed amitotically, although some may perhaps be derived from the endometrial stroma. The syncytial masses project into, and frequently partly surround ("eat their way into"), the uterine stroma, giving the surface of the trophoblast a lobulated appearance. In only rare instances are vacuoles found in the syncytiotrophoblast, and they contain no maternal blood (No. 8020). Macroscopically, no congestion or hemorrhage is visible in the endometrium. Microscopically, the capillary plexus and sinusoids are moderately dilated but contain very few blood cells. It seems that the endometrium itself is adequate for the nourishment of the conceptus at this stage.

It has been found (in Nos. 8020 and 8225) that "the course of several capillaries can be followed through the syncytiotrophoblast. The endothelial walls of the capillaries are intact to the point where each vessel enters and leaves the trophoblast, but between these points red blood cells can be seen to occupy a series of irregularly shaped spaces, which are in continuity with one another" (Harris and Ramsey, 1966). These spaces, however, "are unlike the well-rounded vacuoles occasionally observed in syncytiotrophoblast," and they are "much smaller

RUS ERINE CAVITY

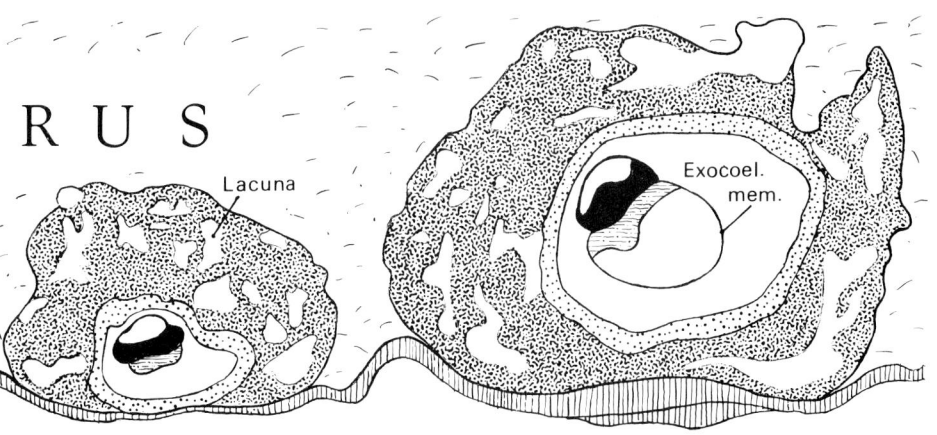

| 5b | 5c |

than the definitive lacunae" present within a couple of days (*ibid.*). It is assumed that "the syncytium advances by a flowing movement that engulfs the blood vessels" in the capillary plexus of the adjacent stratum compactum (*ibid.*). Isolated endothelial cells in the lacunae may lend support to the supposition that capillaries have been engulfed (Dr. Ramsey, personal communication, 1972).

Electron microscopic studies of the rabbit indicate that, in the vicinity of the blastocyst, the uterine epithelium becomes a "symplasma," due to the disintegration of cell membranes (Larsen, 1970). Fusion of the uterine symplasma with the syncytiotrophoblast then takes place, and what are believed to be similar appearances (in No. 8020) have been claimed in the human (*ibid.*).

Extra-embryonic mesoblast. The formation of mesoblast [1] is just beginning, although an exocoelomic membrane has not yet begun to form. Some authors believe that the extra-embryonic mesoblast is developing *in situ* by "delamination" [2] from the cytotrophoblast (Hertig and Rock, 1945 and 1949), although contributions by migration from the endoderm are by no means excluded (*ibid.*). Until further information becomes available, several possible sources of origin of the extra-embryonic mesoblast in the

[1] The term "mesoblast," which will be used here, is preferred by Hertig and Rock (1941) to "mesenchyme" ("rather nonspecific"), "primitive mesoderm" ("one might unintentionally imply some connection with the embryonic mesoderm"), or "magma reticulare" (which "refers to the more mature characteristics of this tissue").

[2] Delamination may be defined as the appearance, without cellular migration, of clefts *in loco* within a mass of cells, followed by the gradual separation of the deeper from the more superficial cells (Pasteels, 1945).

human should be kept in mind: germ disc and/or amniotic ectoderm, cytotrophoblast, and endoderm. This matter will be discussed further under stage 5c.

Amnion. The small space between the embryonic disc and the trophoblast (or within the embryonic disc; see below) represents the beginning of the amniotic cavity. It may communicate with the blastocyst cavity. Either the amnion itself or the amniotic cavity may appear first. Thus, in one instance (No. 8225), a single layer of flattened cells is found attached to the trophoblast although the amniotic cavity is scarcely present. In another case (No. 8155), by contrast, a prominent amniotic cavity (formed by the curved epiblast) is present although amniogenesis has not yet begun (fig. 14). In a third specimen (No. 8020), a small cavity is visible and amniogenesis is under way (fig. 13). The amniogenic cells, which are stated to be delaminating from the trophoblast dorsal to the embryonic disc (Hertig and Rock, 1945), appear to be in the process of enclosing the amniotic cavity by fusing with the margin of the germ disc. In summary, the roof and lateral walls of the amniotic cavity are, in Hertig's (1968) view, derived from the cytotrophoblast, and the cells are mesoblastic. The floor, however, is constituted by the epiblast.

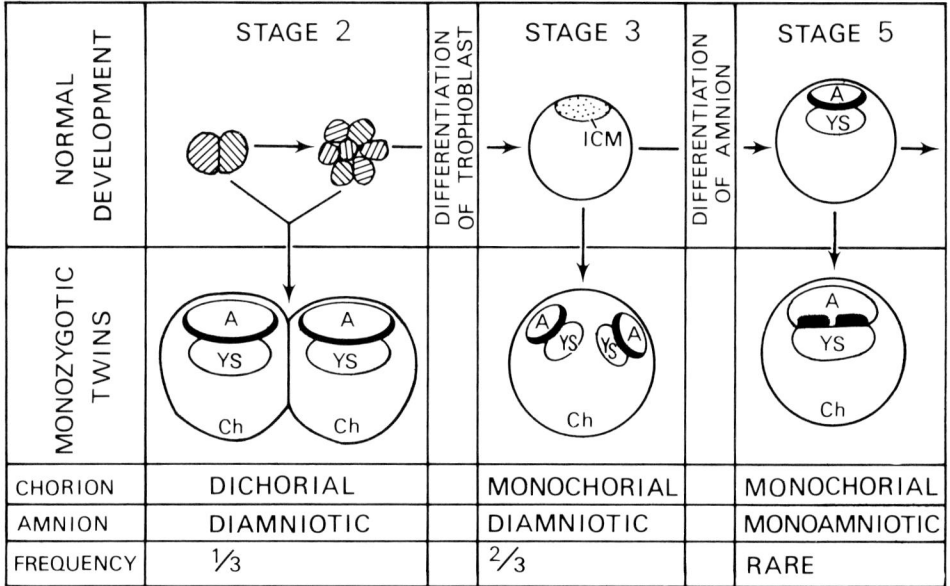

Fig. 10. Diagram to illustrate the presumed mode of development of monozygotic twins in the human. Based partly on Corner (1955). There exist "three critical stages at which the division of the embryo to form monozygotic twins may occur" (Bulmer, 1970). At stage 2, before the differentiation of the trophoblast, separation of the blastomeres would result in twins with separate choria and amnia. At stage 3 (and presumably at stage 4), before differentiation of the amnion, duplication of the inner cell mass would result in twins with a common chorion but separate amnia. At stage 5, duplication of the embryonic disc would result in twins with a common chorion and amnion. Deceptive fusion of the membranes may occur subsequently in certain instances but "the placenta and membranes, if subjected to skilled examination, including microscopic study of the chorionamniotic walls when necessary, will generally yield a correct impression of the type of twinning" (Corner, 1955; see also Allen and Turner, 1971). Partial instead of complete embryonic separation would result in conjoined twins of the various types classified by Wilder (1904).

In general terms, "two distinct methods of amnion formation are ordinarily considered: formation by folding and formation by cavitation, the latter being considered the more specialized" (Mossman, 1937). It seems likely that both of these processes may take part in human amniogenesis, in addition to possible delamination. Recently, a re-examination of the early specimens has led to the conclusion that "a primordial amniotic cavity develops by cavitation within the embryonic knot" at 7½ days, and "there is no clear evidence to support the contention that amniogenic cells arise by delamination from the overlying trophoblast" (Luckett, 1973). That the amniotic cavity arises within the embryonic disc is also the interpretation of Blechschmidt (1968).

The chief function of the amnion is not mechanical protection but rather the enclosing of "the embryonic body in a quantity of liquid sufficient to buoy it up and so allow it to develop symmetrically and freely in all directions" (Mossman, 1937).

Embryonic disc. The term "germ disc" is employed for "the epithelial plate that is derived directly and exclusively from the blastomeric formative cells" (Heuser and Streeter, 1941). The plate may more conveniently be referred to as the epiblast. When the underlying primary endoderm is also included, the term "embryonic disc" (formerly "embryonic shield") is used.

The embryonic disc (figs. 13 and 14) is bilaminar, being composed of the epiblast and the primary endoderm. It is concavoconvex from dorsal to ventral.

The epiblast consists of variably sized, polyhedral cells which either show no precise pattern of arrangement (No. 8020) or are in the form of a pseudostratified columnar epithelium (No. 8155). One or more mitotic figures may be encountered.

The primary endoderm consists of a cap-like mass of small, darkly staining, vesiculated cells without any specific arrangement. Mitotic figures are not seen. As has been mentioned, it is possible that some mesoblastic cells are derived from the endoderm as well as from the trophoblast (Hertig and Rock, 1945).

Specimens of Stage 5a in Carnegie Collection

The "grade" of the specimens listed in Table 9 and the subsequent tables refers to the total grade, including the original quality of a specimen and that subsequent to its handling and preparation in sections.

Specimens of Stage 5a Already Described

Carnegie No. 8225. Described briefly by Hertig and Rock (1945b). Hysterectomy (bicornuate uterus). Anterior wall of uterus. Chorion, 0.33×0.306 mm. Chorionic cavity, 0.228×0.2 mm. Embryonic disc, 0.09×0.078 mm. Perhaps more advanced than No. 8020 (Mazanec, 1959; Harris and Ramsey, 1966), but has also been interpreted as less advanced (Hertig, Rock, and Adams, 1956). Photomicrograph in Hertig, Rock, and Adams (1956; fig. 9). Presumed age, 7 days.

Carnegie No. 8020 (figs. 11-13). Described by Hertig and Rock (1945a). Hysterectomy. Posterior wall of uterus. Chorion, 0.45×0.3 mm. Chorionic cavity, 0.288×0.186 mm. Embryonic disc, 0.126×0.092 mm. New model of blood vessels at implantation site has been prepared (Harris and Ramsey, 1966). Presumed age, 7 days.

A specimen of about 8 days was described briefly by Fruhling, Ginglinger, and Gandar (1954). Curettage. Early

TABLE 9. List of Specimens of Stage 5a in Carnegie Collection*

Serial No.	Grade	Fixative	Cutting Medium	Thinness (micrometers)	Stain	Date and Donor	Reference
8020	Exc.	Alc. & Bouin	C-P	6	H.-E.	1942, A. T. Hertig, Boston, Mass.	Hertig & Rock, 1945a
8155	Exc.	Bouin	C-P	6	H.-E.	1943, A. T. Hertig, Boston, Mass.	Hertig & Rock, 1949
8225	Exc.	Alc. & Bouin	C-P	6	H.-E.	1944, A. T. Hertig, Boston, Mass.	Hertig & Rock, 1945b

*For measurements, see Table 8.

Fig. 11. Surface view of the implantation site of No. 8020, stage 5a, photographed under liquid. The dark ring indicates the chorionic cavity. The opaque area within the ring represents the embryonic mass, that outside the ring represents the trophoblast. The mouths of the endometrial glands appear as dark spots.

Fig. 12. General view of the tissues at and near the implantation site (No. 8020, stage 5a). The edematous endometrium is at the 22nd day of the menstrual cycle. Section 6-5-9.

Fig. 13. Section through the middle of No. 8020, stage 5a. The amniotic cavity and the bilaminar embryonic disc can be seen. The transition from the thin abembryonic trophoblast to the thick, solid layer at the embryonic pole is evident. Large multinucleated masses of syncytiotrophoblast project into the endometrial stroma. A dilated endometrial gland is cut through at the left-hand side of the photomicrograph. Section 6-5-9.

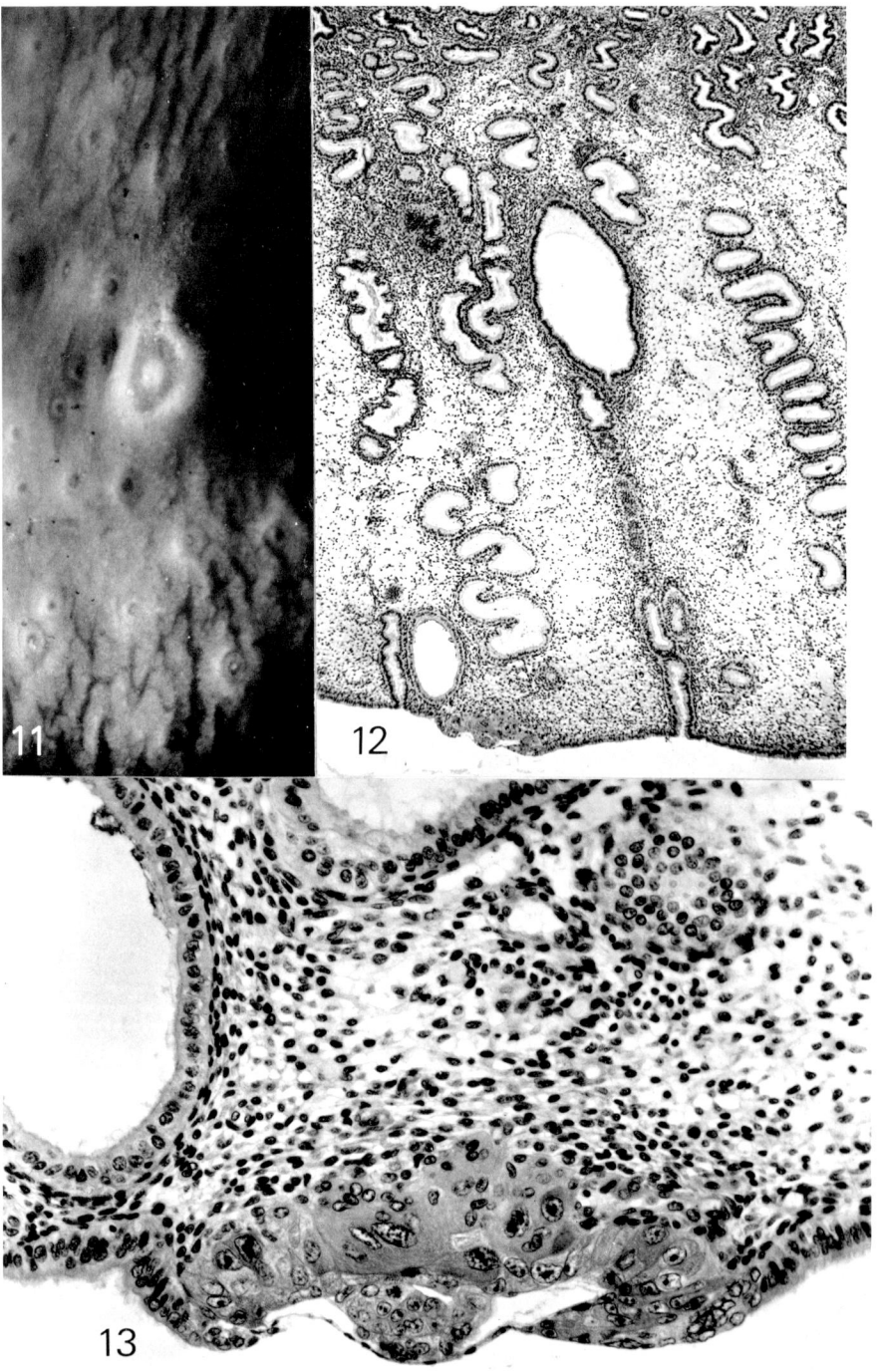

STAGE 5

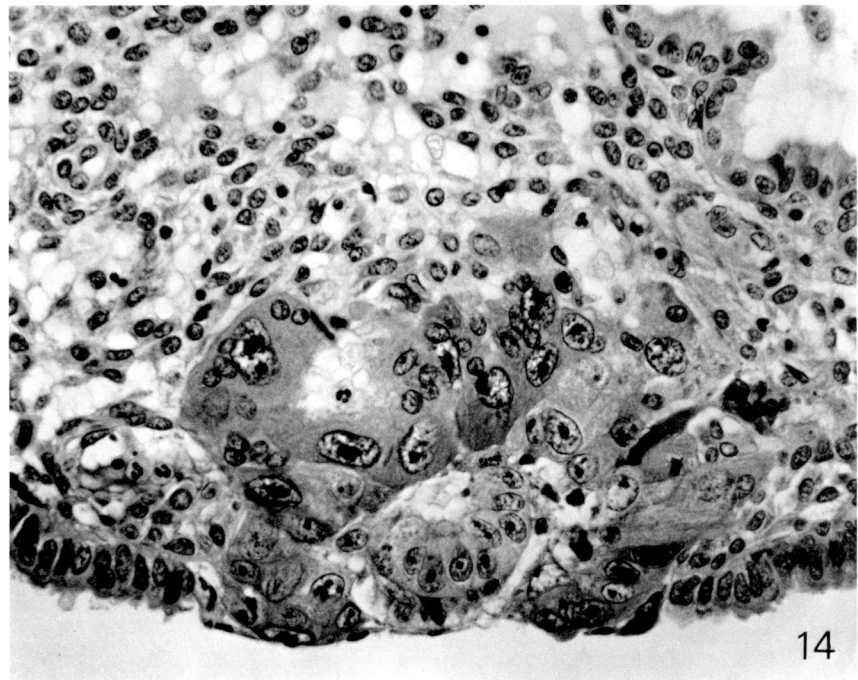

Fig. 14. Section approximately through the middle of No. 8155, stage 5a. The amniotic cavity and the bilaminar embryonic disc can be seen, although amniogenesis has not yet begun. The thick, solid trophoblast at the embryonic pole is mainly syncytiotrophoblast. The endometrial stroma is edematous. Section 4-4-8.

implantation. Few trophoblastic digitations. Beginning amniotic cavity. Most sections through embryonic disc lost.

Carnegie No. 8155 (fig. 14). Described by Hertig and Rock (1949). Hysterectomy. Anterior wall of uterus. Chorion, 0.306 × 0.210 mm. Chorionic cavity, 0.168 × 0.082 mm. Embryonic disc, 0.09 × 0.05 mm.

STAGE 5b

Subdivision 5b is characterized by the appearance of lacunae in the trophoblast (fig. 17). The lacunae communicate with endometrial vessels, and "this joining of maternal vessels to trophoblast is the essence of the uteroplacental circulation of the so-called hemochorial type" (Hertig, 1968). It may be pointed out in passing that "the normal mammalian placenta is defined as an apposition or fusion of the fetal membranes to the uterine mucosa for physiological exchange" (Mossman, 1937).

Amniogenesis is well under way, and the exocoelomic membrane is developed to a variable degree. The chorion attains approximately 0.6 mm in its greatest diameter and hence is readily visible to the naked eye. The space outlined by the internal surface of the chorion is slightly flattened but is undergoing distension. The embryo is about 9 days old, and the embryonic disc is approximately 0.1 mm in diameter.

Endometrium. The endometrial stroma shows an early decidual (commonly called "predecidual") reaction.[3] The conceptus is imperfectly covered by the uterine epithelium. In one specimen (No. 8171), "moderate numbers of leucocytes in the predecidual stroma immediately surrounding" the specimen were noted (Hertig and Rock, 1949). These cells, because of their absence elsewhere, were interpreted as a physiological response to the conceptus. They were "mainly lymphocytes, with lesser numbers of macrophages and polymorphonuclear neutrophils" (*ibid.*).

Trophoblast. Although much of the trophoblast at the embryonic pole and at the equator is of the syncytial variety, an irregular inner rim of cytotrophoblast is present. In places, this rim has begun to form small, discrete masses (cytotrophoblastic clumps) which project into the syncytiotrophoblast and may be regarded as an indication of the future chorionic villi (fig. 25).

Various stages in the formation of lacunae within the syncytiotrophoblast are found (fig. 17). Most of these spaces have coalesced and, at several points, have entered into continuity with the dilated endometrial sinusoids. Few blood cells are seen in either the lacunae or the adjacent sinusoids, however, so that a uteroplacental circulation has scarcely been established. Rather, an ooze into the chorion occurs until chorionic villi appear at a later stage.

The origin of the lacunae has been investigated in the rabbit with the aid of

[3] According to Krafka (1941), "the decidual reaction is generally defined as the appearance of certain large, clear, epithelioid, vesiculated cells, 40 to 50 μ in diameter, ovoid or polyhedral in form, tightly compressed against one another (owing to imbibition of edema fluid or to storage of glycogen), having a conceded origin from the typical fusiform stroma cells primarily in the compacta." The cells are not peculiar to the uterus (they may be found at tubal or ovarian implantation sites, for example), and hence the term "stroma" (better, "stromal") reaction is preferred by Krafka.

electron microscopy. The study revealed "numerous vesicles in the cytoplasm of the syncytial trophoblast. These are the forerunners of larger cavities, approximately 30–40 μm in diameter," which "by their confluence are later transformed into the lacunae of the definitive placenta" (Larsen, 1970). When the trophoblast penetrates the maternal vessels, the lacunae gain access to maternal blood (*ibid.*). The important work of Harris and Ramsey (1966), however, has already been mentioned. According to these latter authors, "during the initial stages of implantation in the human it appears that the syncytiotrophoblast engulfs the capillary plexus in the adjacent *stratum compactum*. It is suggested that part of the plexus remains within the trophoblastic plate as a series of small spaces, which maintain continuity with the maternal circulation and subsequently enlarge to form the lacunae."

Extra-embryonic mesoblast. The mesoblast, which continues to develop, is discussed under stages 5a and 5c.

Amnion. The amniotic cavity, which is smaller than the yolk sac, is almost closed by the amniogenic cells. These cells are stated to be arising *in situ* (as in stage 5a) by delamination from adjacent cytotrophoblast (Hertig and Rock, 1941 and 1949).

Embryonic disc. The bilaminar embryonic disc (fig. 17) resembles that seen at stage 5a.

The epiblast is a pseudostratified columnar epithelium in which the cytoplasm is beginning to become vacuolated ventrally.

The primary endoderm consists of either a single layer or a cap-like mass of cuboidal or polyhedral cells.

Yolk sac. The exocoelomic membrane is attached at the margin of the embryonic disc. The exocoelomic vesicle enclosed by the disc and the membrane of the same name "was first described and figured by Stieve (1931, 1936) in the Werner [5c] embryo, although he did not name it as such; he referred to it as the 'Dottersackanlage,' and, though he frequently referred to the 'Dottersack,' he made it clear that the vesicle is not the definitive yolk-sac as usually described" (Davies, 1944).

The exocoelomic membrane was described in the macaque as an "intrachorionic mesothelial membrane" that "must be regarded as a part of the primitive mesoblast" (Heuser, 1932). In a later publication, however, the wall of the primary yolk sac of the macaque was stated either to be derived from endodermal cells "which spread to line the chorion," or to "arise by delamination from the trophoblast" (Heuser and Streeter, 1941). Elsewhere in the same article, the exocoelomic membrane is said to be derived either by delamination from the endoderm (misprinted as "endothelium") or "by creeping in from the sides as a spreading membrane" of mesoblast.

In the human, the exocoelomic membrane (together with the disc) encloses the primary yolk sac cavity, and may perhaps be arising *in situ* by delamination from the adjacent cytotrophoblast (Hertig and Rock, 1945a and 1949) although its origin is by no means clear. A similar mode of origin has been proposed for the scattered mesoblastic cells that are found between the trophoblast and the exocoelomic membrane (Hertig and Rock, 1949).

The trophoblast with its mesoblastic lining may now be called the chorion (Hamilton and Boyd, 1950). The term "chorion" is commonly used "for the outer fetal membrane made up of trophoblast and somatic mesoderm" (Mossman, 1937), whether it be avascular (e.g., the "true chorion" of the pig) or vascular (e.g., the allanto-chorion of the human).

SPECIMENS OF STAGE 5b IN CARNEGIE COLLECTION

These are listed in Table 10.

SPECIMENS OF STAGE 5b ALREADY DESCRIBED

Carnegie No. 8171. Described by Hertig and Rock (1949). Hysterectomy. Posterior wall of uterus. Abnormal leucocytic infiltration of endometrium. Chorion, 0.422 × 0.404 mm. Chorionic cavity, 0.164 × 0.138 mm. Embryonic disc, 0.114 × 0.088 mm. A cellular remnant within the yolk sac, because it is probably derived from the endoderm, "may, in a sense, be regarded as an abnormal form of twin embryo" (*ibid.*). Presumed age, 9 days.

Carnegie No. 8215. Described briefly by Hertig and Rock (1945c). Hysterectomy. Posterior wall of uterus. Chorion, 0.525 × 0.498 mm. Chorionic cavity, 0.228 × 0.21 mm. Embryonic disc, 0.084 × 0.052 mm. Lacunae perhaps further developed than in No. 8171 (Mazanec, 1959) but specimen has been "considered to be slightly younger . . . because the decidual reaction is not yet apparent" (Hertig, Rock, and Adams, 1956). Photomicrographs in Hertig, Rock, and Adams (1956; figs. 15 and 17). Presumed age, 9 days.

Carnegie No. 8004 (figs. 15–17). Described by Hertig and Rock (1945a). Hysterectomy. Posterior wall of uterus. Chorion, 0.582 × 0.45 mm. Chorionic cavity, 0.312 × 0.185 mm. Embryonic disc, 0.132 × 0.1 mm.

Carnegie No. 9350. Described briefly by Heuser (1956). Hysterectomy. At junction of posterior and anterior walls. Chorion, 0.59 × 0.58 mm. Chorionic cavity, 0.3 × 0.1 mm. Embryonic disc, 0.132 × 0.09 mm. Presumed age, 9 days.

TABLE 10. List of Specimens of Stage 5b in Carnegie Collection*

Serial No.	Grade	Fixative	Cutting Medium	Thinness (micrometers)	Stain	Date and Donor	Reference
8004	Exc.	Alc. & Bouin	C-P	6	H.-E.	1942, A. T. Hertig, Boston, Mass.	Hertig & Rock, 1945a
8171	Exc.	Alc.	C-P	6	H.-E.	1943, A. T. Hertig, Boston, Mass.	Hertig & Rock, 1949
8215	Exc.	Alc. & Bouin	C-P	6	H.-E.	1944, A. T. Hertig, Boston, Mass.	Hertig & Rock, 1945c
9350	Exc.	Bouin	?	?	H.-E.	1955, C. H. Heuser & R. Torpin, Augusta, Ga.	Heuser, 1956

*For measurements, see Table 8.

STAGE 5c

In their proposals to subdivide horizon V, Hertig, Rock, and Adams (1956) distinguished 5b, "formation of trophoblastic lacunae with amniotic and exocoelomic cavities," from 5c, "intercommunicating lacunae with beginning utero-lacunar circulation." In 5b, "although the vast majority of the lacunar spaces have coalesced they contain relatively little maternal blood, and that mostly plasma, since few adjacent capillary sinusoids of the endometrial stroma communicate directly with the lacunar network as yet." In 5c, "the lacunar spaces now intercommunicate and contain enough maternal blood" to enable specimens at this stage to be "easily identified on careful gross examination of the endometrial surface prior to fixation. Such lacunar blood appears as a discontinuous red circle about 1 mm in diameter" (fig. 20).

Because the quantitative changes between 5b and 5c may prove difficult to discern, and because a given specimen may not have been examined grossly prior to fixation, it was at first considered that the two substages should be combined here into one for reasons of practicality. Nevertheless, in order to avoid complicating further an already established system, and in order to continue the subdivision of an otherwise large and prolonged (four day) group of embryos, it has been decided to retain 5b and 5c. It is hoped that, perhaps by comparing the measurements and the appearances of a given specimen in section with the photomicrographs of embryos already staged, it may be possible to assign new examples to their appropriate place. If not, they should be classified as merely stage 5.

Stage 5c, then, is characterized by the intercommunication of the lacunae. Moreover, the contained blood is sufficient to appear as a discontinuous red ring, so that identification of the conceptus is possible on careful gross examination of the endometrial surface prior to fixation (fig. 20). Embryos of stage 5c are believed to be 11 to 12 days old, the chorion measures about 0.75 to 1 mm in its greatest diameter, and the embryonic disc is approximately 0.15 to 0.2 mm in diameter. The space outlined by the internal surface of the chorion now appears distended again.

The availability of human specimens, after reaching its lowest point at stage 4, increases greatly with the advent of stage 5c, and from now onwards the account will be confined almost entirely to the human.

Endometrium. The endometrial stroma around the conceptus again shows an early decidual ("predecidual") reaction, and indeed decidua may be said to be present. The uterine epithelium continues its repair of the defect and, within the defect, a fibrinous, leucocytic, hemorrhagic coagulum may be present.[4] Moreover, a "constant attempt on the part of maternal tissues to heal the endometrium persists until . . . the conceptus is of six weeks' developmental age" (Hertig, 1968).

---

[4] The operculum, or closing plate, according to Krafka (1941), "is generally described as a simple organizing clot, including fibrin, fibrinoid, living and necrotic leucocytes, old and recent hemorrhage, and degenerating stroma." That it is something more than a simple organizing clot, however, is indicated by the circumstance that "both the aperture and the operculum increase in size" (*ibid.*). The nomenclature of this region (which includes a number of German terms, such as *Verschlusspfropf, Schlusscoagulum,* and *Gewebspilz*) has been clarified by Hamilton and Gladstone (1942), who defined the operculum deciduae (of Teacher, 1925) as the flattened or dome-shaped head of the fungus- or mushroom-shaped structure, and the occlusion- or closing-plug as the part occupying and closing the aperture of entry.

Fig. 15. Surface view of the implantation site of No. 8004, stage 5b, photographed under liquid. The dark area in the middle represents the abembryonic wall of the specimen.

Fig. 16. General view of the tissues at and near the implantation site (No. 8004, stage 5b). The "predecidual" endometrium is at the 26th day of the menstrual cycle. Section 11-4-4.

Fig. 17. Section through the middle of No. 8004, stage 5b. Some epithelial regeneration of the endometrium has taken place over the specimen. The large mass of syncytiotrophoblast shows intercommunicating lacunae. The chorionic cavity is surrounded by a thin layer of cytotrophoblast. The amniotic cavity and the bilaminar embryonic disc can be seen. Section 11-4-5.

STAGE 5

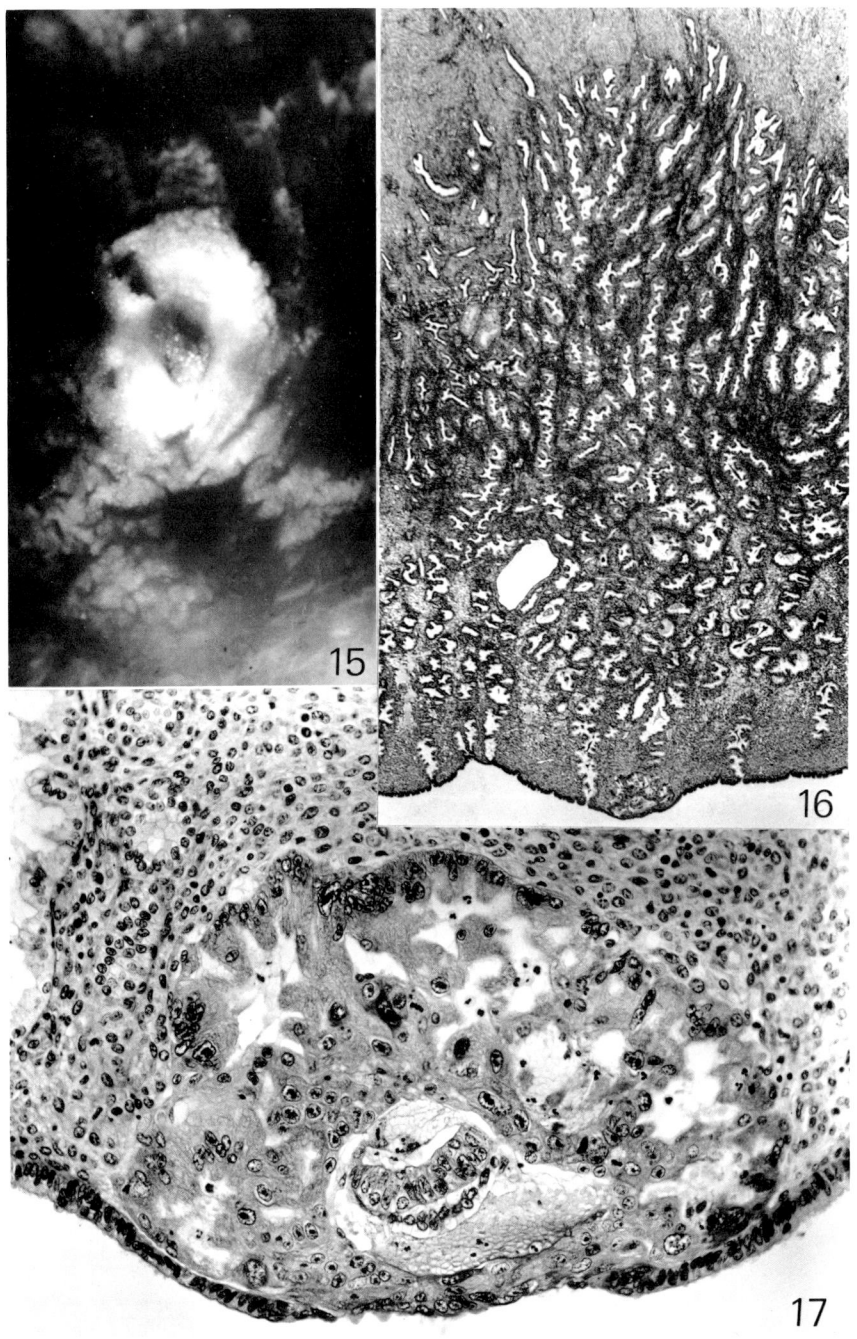

Chorion. The cytotrophoblast, although it varies in thickness, is generally formed by a single layer of cuboidal cells. Masses of proliferating cytotrophoblast project into the syncytiotrophoblast. These cytotrophoblastic clumps (Davies, 1944), seen already at stage 5b, may be regarded as an indication of the future chorionic villi (fig. 25). In a few instances (in No. 7700) the beginning of a mesoblastic and angioblastic core has been detected. Such appearances may conveniently be termed mesoblastic crests (Krafka, 1941).

The syncytiotrophoblast forms about three-fourths of the total trophoblastic shell. It contains large, irregular, intercommunicating lacunae lined by a brush border and containing an increasing amount of maternal blood. The filling of the lacunae may result in a brilliant red circle (fig. 20) which enables the implantation site to be identified before fixation (Hertig, 1968). The presence of the lacunae gives the syncytiotrophoblast a sponge-like structure, and the lacunar system is primarily labyrinthine (Hamilton and Boyd, 1960). The implantation area presents intercommunicating capillaries, which, by several relatively large branches, communicate directly with the lacunae within the trophoblast. Also within the syncytiotrophoblast are found what appear to be phagocytosed maternal blood cells and possibly other tissues.

According to Park (1957), sex chromatin is absent up to 12 days, that is, during the first five stages. In one (abnormal) specimen (No. 8000) of 5c, an incidence of less than one per cent was found in the trophoblast.

Extra-embryonic mesoblast. In addition to the continuing formation of mesoblast (from the cytotrophoblast, according to Hertig and Rock, 1941), angiogenesis is beginning at the abembryonic pole, where angioblastic cells seem to be delaminating from the cytotrophoblast (*ibid.*).

The origin of the extra-embryonic mesoblast has already been touched on under stage 5a. This tissue appears before the primitive streak is formed, and its origin is still subject to discussion. In his study of the Miller (5c) specimen, Streeter (1926) concluded that the primary mesoblast "must have either separated off from the inner cell mass during the formation of the segmentation cavity or have been derived from the trophoblast. Since it is, in reality, so largely concerned in the differentiation of the trophoblastic structures, the latter is the more probable explanation." From his investigations of the same specimen and more particularly of macaque embryos, Hertig (1935) believed in the "simultaneous origin of angioblasts and primary mesoderm by a process of delamination and differentiation from the chorionic trophoblast. . . ."

On the other hand, Hill's (1932) studies of the Primate embryo led him to believe in "the existence in early embryos of the Pithecoid and man of a mesodermal proliferating area involving the postero-median margin of the shield-ectoderm and the immediately adjoining portion of the amniotic ectoderm which contributes to, if it does not entirely form, the connecting stalk primordium. This proliferating area, it may be suggested, functionally replaces, if it does not actually represent, the hinder end of the primitive streak of the Tarsioid and the Lemuroid. . . ." In pursuance of this idea, Florian (1933) concluded that, in the Werner (5c) embryo, an "area of fusion of the ectoderm of the caudal part of the embryonic shield with the primary mesoderm" was a site where "at least a part of the primary mesoderm originates."

This theory of Hill and Florian, supported recently by Luckett (1971), has been rather neglected in human embryology. It should be kept in mind, however, that the theory of trophoblastic delamination and that of a mesoblastic proliferating area are not necessarily mutually exclusive. It is possible that the extra-embryonic mesoblast is being formed by both modes of origin.

Amnion. The amniotic cavity is nearly completely closed (fig. 22), although (in No. 7700) amniogenic cells still appear to be in the process of "being added to by the adjacent trophoblast" (Hertig, 1968, fig. 70). The cells are partly epithelial and partly mesenchymal. The amniotic cavity is still smaller than the yolk sac.

Embryonic disc. The bilaminar embryonic disc (fig. 22) resembles that seen at stage 5b. It is either basically circular on dorsal view, so that a longitudinal axis is not yet evident (No. 7699), or it is pyriform or ovoid, so that an apparent axis may be more or less envisioned (No. 7700 and No. 8139). It is possible also that a condensation of extra-embryonic mesoblast may serve to indicate the caudal end of the disc (Hertig, Rock, and Adams, 1956, fig. 38).

The epiblast is a pseudostratified columnar epithelium in which vacuoles are seen, mostly ventrally. Some mitotic figures may be observed.

The primary endoderm is sharply demarcated peripherally from the adjoining cells of the exocoelomic membrane. Mitotic figures, if found at all, are rare.

Yolk sac. The exocoelomic membrane (fig. 21), which was first figured by Stieve (1931) in the Werner embryo, is clearly formed, although it may be deficient in places.

SPECIMENS OF STAGE 5c IN CARNEGIE COLLECTION

These are listed in Table 11.

SPECIMENS OF STAGE 5c ALREADY DESCRIBED

Davies-Harding. Described by Davies (1944). Hysterectomy. Anterior wall of uterus. Incomplete (almost one-half of embryonic disc missing). "No true villi." Exocoelomic membrane present. Extensive extra-embryonic mesoblast. Slightly later stage of development than No. 8004 (Davies, 1944, Addendum), which belongs to 5b. "Possibly pathological" (Boyd and Hamilton, 1970). Chorion, 1.18×0.55 mm. Chorionic cavity, 0.409×0.238 mm. Embryonic disc, 0.117 mm. May be regarded as transitional between 5b and 5c. Presumed age, 9 or 10 days.

Carnegie No. 7699. Described by Hertig and Rock (1941). Hysterectomy. Posterior wall of uterus. Chorion, 1.026×0.713 mm. Chorionic cavity, 0.48×0.336 mm. Embryonic disc, 0.138×0.138 mm. New model of blood vessels at implantation site has been prepared (Harris and Ramsey, 1966). Presumed age, 11 days.

Carnegie No. 4900, Miller. Described by Streeter (1926). Curettage. Angiogenesis described by Hertig (1935). Incomplete (some sections missing). Exocoelomic membrane present. New graphic reconstruction made by Streeter (1939, a and b). Chorion, 0.9 mm. Chorionic cavity, 0.4 mm. Presumed age, 10–11 days or perhaps even 12 days (Krafka, 1941).

Dible-West. Described by Dible and West (1941). Autopsy. Posterior wall of uterus. Incomplete. Chorionic cavity, 0.47×0.28 mm. Embryonic disc, 0.1×0.02 mm. Presumed age, 11–13 days.

TABLE 11. List of Specimens of Stage 5c in Carnegie Collection*

Serial No.	Grade	Fixative	Cutting Medium	Thinness (micrometers)	Stain	Date and Donor	Remarks and Reference
4900	Poor	?	P	10	?	1925, J. W. Miller, Barmen, Germany	Incomplete. Streeter, 1926
7699	Exc.	Bouin	C-P	6	H.-E.	1939, A. T. Hertig, Boston, Mass.	Hertig & Rock, 1941
7700	Exc.	Bouin	C-P	6	H.-E.	1938, A. T. Hertig, Boston, Mass.	Hertig & Rock, 1941
7770	Exc.	Bouin	C-P	6 & 10	H.-E.	1940, A. T. Hertig, Boston, Mass.	Abnormal
7771	Exc.	Bouin	C-P	10	H.-E.	1940, A. T. Hertig, Boston, Mass.	Abnormal
7950	Exc.	Alc. & Bouin	C-P	6	H.-E.	1941, A. T. Hertig, Boston, Mass.	Hertig & Rock, 1944
8000	Poor	Alc. & Bouin	C-P	8	H.-E.	1942, A. T. Hertig, Boston, Mass.	Abnormal
8139	Exc.	?	C-P	6	H.-E.	1943, A. Marchetti, New York, N.Y.	Incomplete. Marchetti, 1945
8299	Exc.	Alc. & Bouin	C-P	6	H.-E. phlox.	1945, A. T. Hertig, Boston, Mass.	Abnormal
8329	Exc.	Alc. & Bouin	C-P	6	H.-E. phlox.	1945, A. T. Hertig, Boston, Mass.	Abnormal
8330	Exc.	Alc. & Bouin	C-P	6	H.-E. phlox.	1945, A. T. Hertig, Boston, Mass.	
8370	Poor	Alc. & Bouin	C-P	6	H.-E.	1946, A. T. Hertig, Boston, Mass.	Abnormal
8558	Exc.	Alc. & Bouin	C-P	6	H.-E.	1947, A. T. Hertig, Boston, Mass.	

*For measurements, see Table 8.

An autopsy specimen was described by Müller (1930). Only one section near embryonic disc.

A specimen was described by Wilson (1954). Endometrial biopsy. Chorion, 0.5 × 0.6 mm. Chorionic cavity, 0.47 × 0.24 mm. Between the amnion and the cytotrophoblast, "a small accumulation of fibroblastic cells . . . probably represents the earliest stage of the Bauchstiel." The endoderm is being "delaminated from the embryonic disc." Imperfectly developed exocoelomic membrane. Presumed age, 11 days.

Carnegie No. 7950. Described briefly by Hertig and Rock (1944). Chorion, 0.75 × 0.45 mm. Chorionic cavity, 0.4 × 0.26 mm. Embryonic disc, 0.16 × 0.07 mm. Slightly more developed than No. 7699, although embryo is a little less differentiated. Photomicrographs in Hertig, Rock, and Adams (1956; figs. 27 and 35). Presumed age, 12 days.

Carnegie No. 7700 (figs. 18–22). Described by Hertig and Rock (1941). Hysterectomy. Posterior wall of uterus. Chorion, 0.948 × 0.835 mm. Chorionic cavity, 0.55 × 0.498 mm. Embryonic disc, 0.204 × 0.165 mm. Presumed age, 12 days.

Carnegie No. 8558. Measurements and photomicrographs in Hertig, Rock, and Adams (1956; figs. 30 and 37). Chorion, 0.96 × 0.52 mm. Chorionic cavity, 0.58 × 0.36 mm. Embryonic disc, 0.22 × 0.08 mm. Presumed age, 12 days.

Carnegie No. 8330. Measurements and photomicrographs in Hertig, Rock, and Adams (1956; figs. 30 and 37). Chorion, 0.85 × 0.65 mm. Chorionic cavity, 0.46 × 0.4 mm. Embryonic disc, 0.216 × 0.063 mm. Condensation of extra-embryonic mesoblast perhaps indicates "the beginning of axis formation" (*ibid.*). Presumed age, 12 days.

Kleinhans. Described by Grosser (1922). Autopsy. Only one section; embryonic disc not seen. Chorion, 0.8 × 0.65 mm. Chorionic cavity, 0.35 × 0.15 mm.

Barnes. Described by Hamilton, Barnes, and Dodds (1943), and further by Hamilton and Boyd (1960). Hysterectomy. Posterior wall of uterus. Pathological edema in endometrium (Davies, 1944). Chorion, 0.931 × 0.77 × 0.737 mm. Presumed age, 10–11 days or perhaps 12 days (Davies, 1944).

Werner (Prof. Werner Gerlach). Described by Stieve (1936), with graphic reconstruction by Florian. Autopsy. Chorion, 0.78 × 1.36 × 0.72 mm. Embryonic disc, 0.18 × 0.12 mm. Some large, round cells in the epiblast are mentioned as possible primordial germ cells. Extra-embryonic coelom and primordia (mesoblastic crests) of chorionic villi (Hertig and Rock, 1941). "Connecting stalk," very indistinct. Rostrocaudal axis (Florian, 1945) but no primitive streak (Florian, 1933). Epiblast fused with extra-embryonic mesoblast caudally (Florian, 1933) and perhaps is origin of latter (Florian, 1945). Perhaps 12 days.

A specimen described by Dankmeijer and Wielenga (1968) belongs to stage 5. Curettage. Incomplete.

Carnegie No. 8139. Described by Marchetti (1945), who admitted that it is "not entirely normal." Curettage. Chorion, 0.706 × 1.2 mm. Chorionic cavity, 0.635 × 0.582 mm. Embryonic disc, 0.126 × 0.048 × 0.116 mm. Embryo located centrally in chorionic cavity, which is filled with mesoblast. Embryonic disc, slightly ovoid, i.e., presents a longitudinal axis. Described originally as previllous, although "primitive villi" (stage 6) are mentioned by Boyd and Hamilton (1970): folds of undulating contour of cytotrophoblast are not yet

Fig. 18. Surface view of the implantation site of No. 7700, stage 5c.

Fig. 19. Side view of the implantation site of No. 7700, stage 5c.

Fig. 20. View of the implantation site of No. 7700, stage 5c, as seen in the cleared celloidin block. The irregular, dark ring is due to maternal blood within the trophoblastic lacunae, and is a characteristic feature of subdivision 5c as it has been defined by Hertig, Rock, and Adams (1956).

STAGE 5

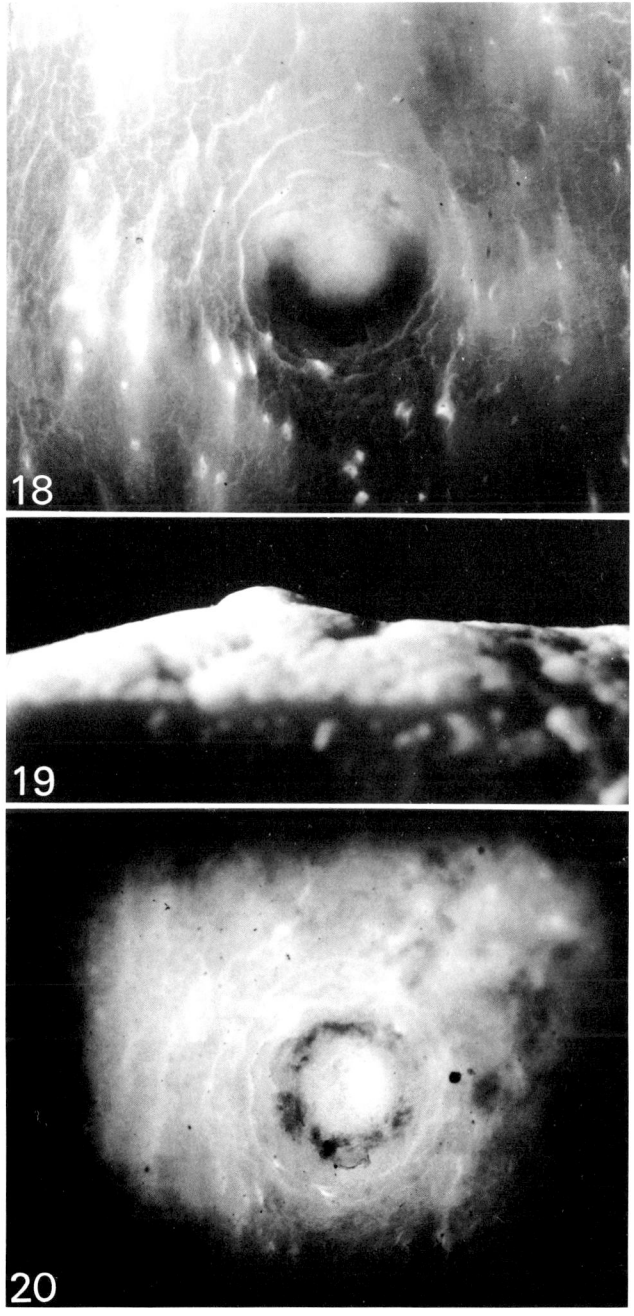

Fig. 21. Section through the middle of No. 7700, stage 5c. The space outlined by the internal surface of the chorion now appears distended again. However, a gradient of differentiating trophoblast from abembryonic to embryonic pole is still evident. Intercommunicating lacunae are visible in the syncytiotrophoblast. Extra-embryonic mesoblast, the exocoelomic membrane, and the yolk sac can be seen. The endometrial stroma is edematous and decidua is developing. Section 6-1-5.

Fig. 22. The bilaminar embryonic disc of No. 7700, stage 5c. The amnion overlying the disc is not yet complete. The epiblast is a pseudostratified columnar epithelium. The surrounding cytotrophoblast is evident, and lacunae can be seen in the syncytiotrophoblast. Cytotrophoblastic clumps may be regarded as an indication of the future chorionic villi. Section 6-1-5.

STAGE 5

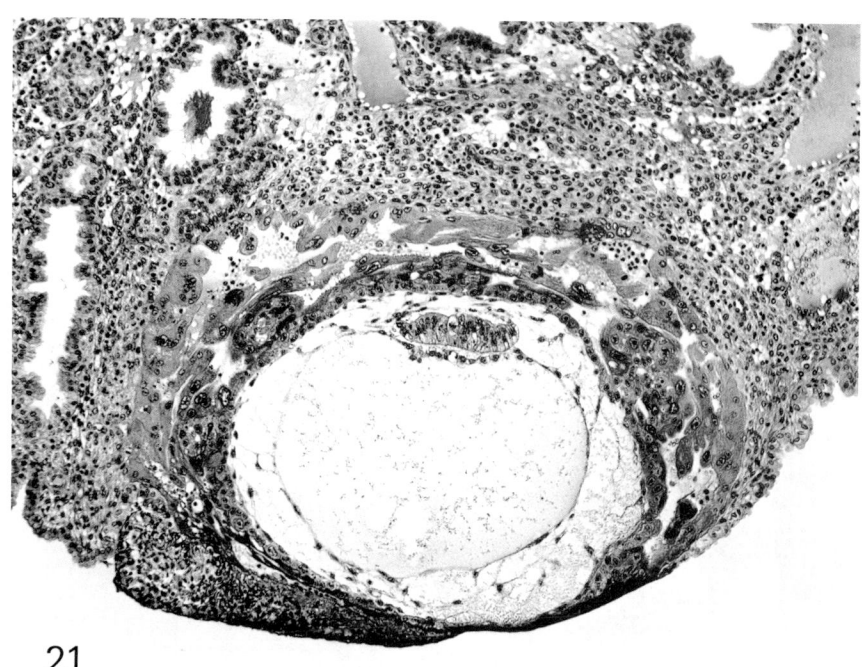

21

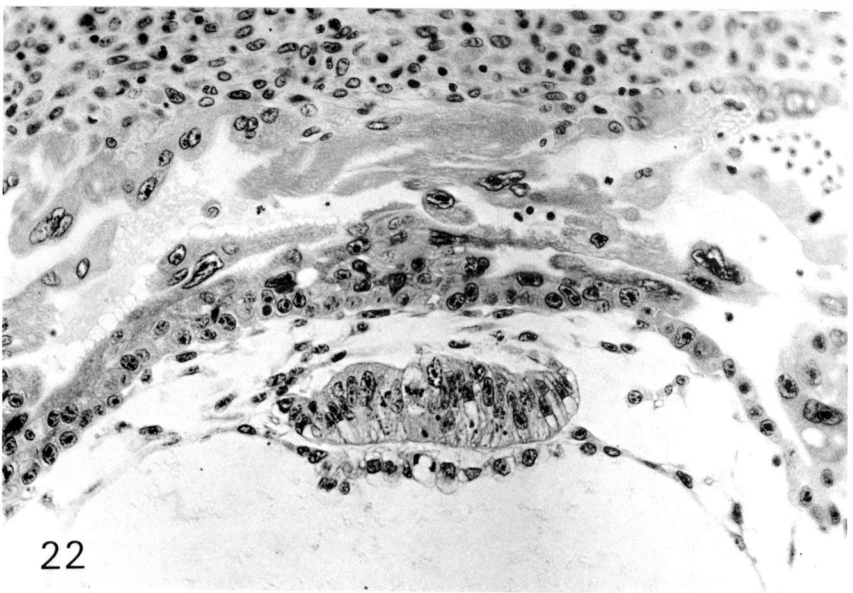

22

"primitive unbranching villi, although they may be the primordia of them" (Marchetti, 1945; see fig. 5). Yolk sac present. May be regarded as transitional between stages 5 and 6. Presumed age, 13 days.

A specimen noted by Bandler (1912) was embedded in tubal mucosa and showed "as yet absolutely no suggestion of chorionic villi." No details available.

A specimen described by Pommerenke (1958) belongs to stage 5. Curettage. Incomplete. Embryo not included.

Macafee. Described by Morton (1949). Curettage. Probably belongs to stage 5. Embryonic disc not found.

A specimen described by Scipiades (1938) belongs either to stage 5 or to stage 6, probably the former, "but its preservation is so poor that accurate conclusions are impossible" (Hertig and Rock, 1941). Curettage. Chorion, 1.498 × 0.49 mm. Chorionic cavity, 0.99 mm. Embryonic disc (only two sections available), 0.18 × 0.048 mm. Presumed age, 11–12 days.

A specimen featured by Thomas and van Campenhout (1963) probably belongs to stage 5, although some trophoblastic thickenings of a villous character were said to be present.

Teacher-Bryce I. A pathological specimen of stage 5 described by Bryce (1924).

Sch. (Schönig). A pathological specimen of stage 5 described by von Möllendorff (1921).

A pathological specimen described by Keller and Keller (1954) was embedded in the stroma of the ostium uteri.

Several pathological specimens of stage 5c are in the Carnegie Collection. Nos. 8370, 7770, 8299 (malpositioned embryonic disc, Hertig, 1968, fig. 132), 8329, 8000 (superficial implantation), and 7771 (no embryo) have been measured and illustrated by Hertig, Rock, and Adams (1956).

STAGE 6

Stage 6 is characterized by the first appearance of chorionic villi (fig. 30), which almost immediately begin to branch. The maximum diameter of the chorion varies from 1 to 4.5 mm, that of its enclosed cavity from 0.6 to 4.5 mm. The embryonic disc varies from 0.15 to 0.5 mm in maximum diameter, and the age is believed to be about 13 days.

The space bounded by the internal surface of the chorion begins to expand greatly towards the end of stage 5 and during stage 6 (fig. 23).

Axial features are not evident, or at least have not been described, in all stage 6 embryos. Moreover, in some instances, their presence is in dispute. It is possible, however, were the fixation and plane of section always suitable, were the series complete and free from distortion, and were an adequate search made, that axial features would be found. Thus, in the well-known Peters specimen, which is frequently considered as not yet showing axial features, the possible presence of an allantois was raised originally (Peters, 1899), and apparently Grosser believed for a time that a primitive streak was present.

Hence it is convenient to distinguish (a) those embryos in which little or no axial differentiation has occurred, or at least has not been noted, from (b) those embryos in which axial features, particularly a primitive streak, have definitely been recorded (fig. 32). This distinction corresponds more or less to Mazanec's (1959) groups V and VI, respectively. In the latter, according to Mazanec, the chorionic villi have already begun to branch.

It may be of interest to mention that those specimens (referred to here as 6a) in which definite axial features have not been described are characterized by a slightly smaller chorion (1–3 mm, as compared with 2–4.5 mm in the remainder, 6b), contained cavity (0.6–2.2 mm, as compared with 1.3–4.5 mm), and embryonic disc (0.15–0.22 mm, as compared with 0.15–0.5 mm).

A chart indicating the derivation of various tissues and structures is presented as figure 24.

The writer is indebted to Dr. J. E. Jirásek, of Prague, for helpful suggestions concerning the delimitation of stages 6 to 8.

Decidua. The decidua (fig. 30) varies considerably in thickness at the implantation site but is generally between 3 and 12 mm (Krafka, 1941). A decidual reaction is present, a variable amount of edema and leucocytic infiltration is found, and actively secreting glands and prominent blood vessels are noticeable. Compact, spongy, and basal strata are distinguishable from superficial to deep (*ibid.*). At about this time the well-known subdivision of the decidua into three topographical components may be employed: (a) the decidua basalis is that situated at the deepest (embryonic) pole of the conceptus; (b) the decidua capsularis is reflected over the rest of the chorionic sac; and (c) the decidua parietalis lines the uterine cavity except at the site of implantation.

Chorion. The increasing structural complexity of the trophoblast from superficial to lateral and basal aspects has been attributed by Ramsey (1938) to the more advantageous nutritive conditions prevailing at the latter sites. The coalescence of the lacunae forms the intervillous space, which, placed as an offshoot

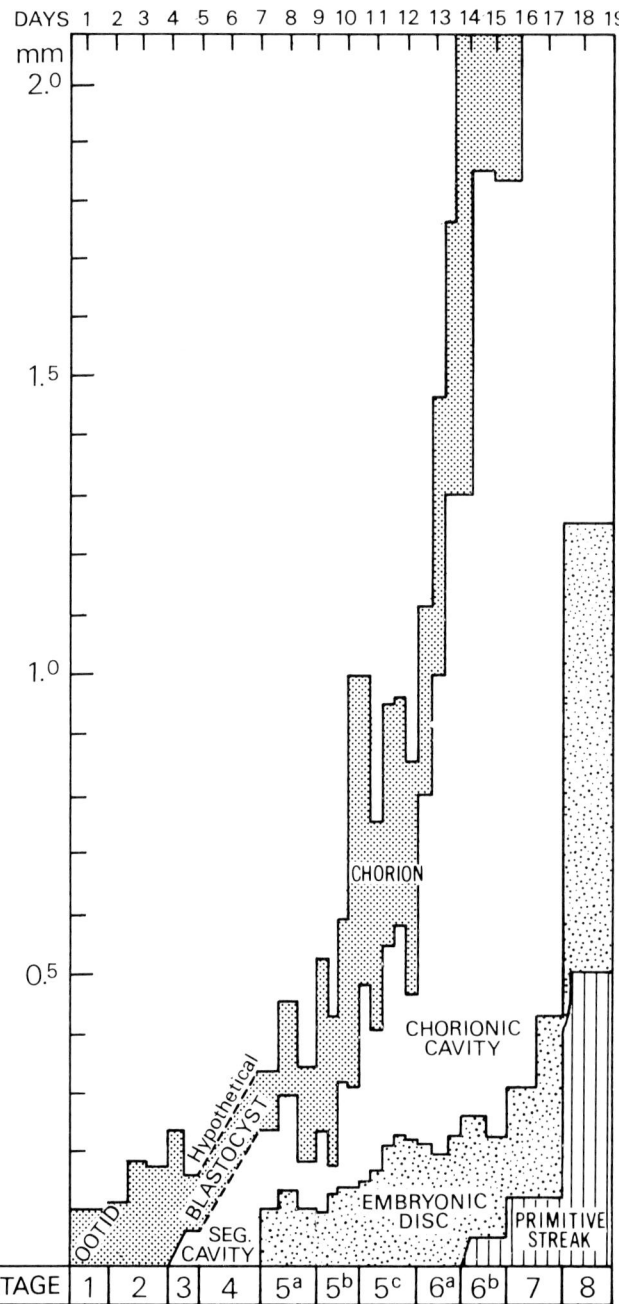

Fig. 23. Graph to show the progression in size from stage 1 to stage 8. Based on the measurements of 28 specimens. The interrupted lines indicate hypothetical values for stage 4. An enormous expansion of the chorionic cavity begins to take place towards the end of stage 5.

STAGE 6

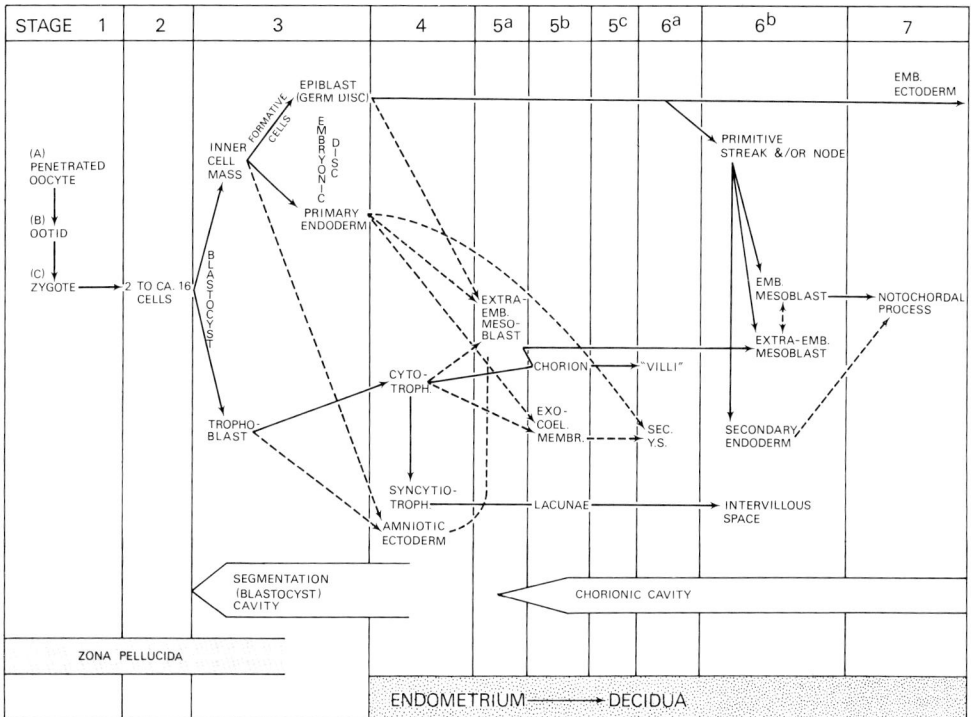

Fig. 24. Chart to show main derivations of various tissues and structures during the first seven stages. Less certain and disputed derivations are indicated by interrupted lines.

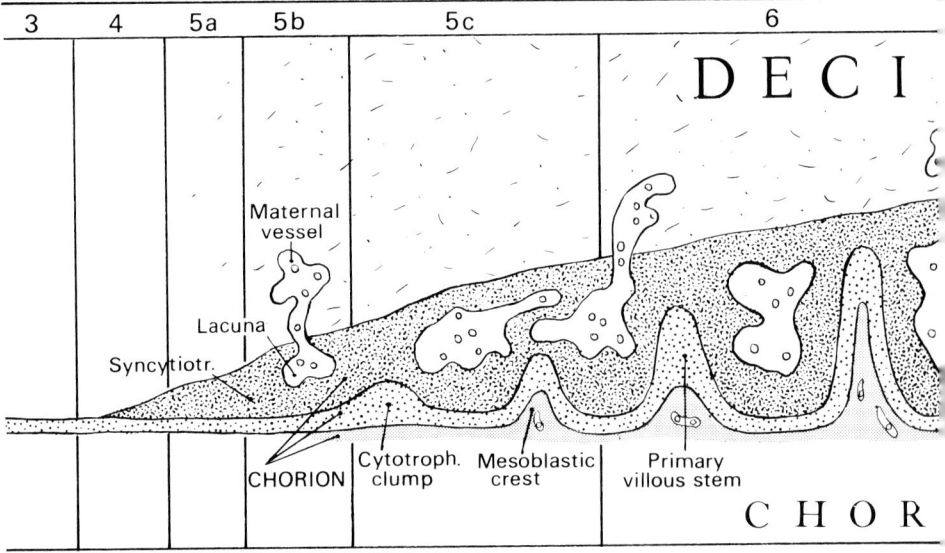

Fig. 25. Highly simplified scheme to show the preliminary events during stages 3 to 7 that lead to the development of the placenta. The cytotrophoblast (stage 3) gives origin to syncytiotrophoblast (stage 4), and lacunae appear in the latter (stage 5b). The appearance of a meso-

on the uterine circulation, may be regarded as "a variety of arteriovenous aneurysm" (Hertig, 1968). The syncytiotrophoblast is more active enzymatically than the cytotrophoblast, and is believed, among other functions, to be responsible for the secretion of chorionic gonadotropin.

The cytotrophoblastic clumps and mesoblastic crests of stage 5 have now progressed to form processes that are commonly known as chorionic villi (fig. 25). Several authors have pointed out that "the initial villi do not arise as free and separate outgrowths from the chorionic plate" into the lacunar spaces (Boyd and Hamilton, 1970). Trophoblastic trabeculae, which initially are syncytial in character, come to possess a central process of cytotrophoblast and are generally termed primary villi. None of the trabeculae, however, possesses a free distal end, because these "primary villous stems" do not arise as individual and separate sprouts from the chorion (Hamilton and Boyd, 1960) but rather by invagination of syncytiotrophoblast (fig. 25).

The mesoblastic crests form the cores of the villi, and the cytotrophoblastic clumps form caps from which cytotrophoblastic columns proceed externally. These columns, indications of which have been seen also at stage 5c, make contact with the stroma and form a border zone (penetration zone, Greenhill, 1927), the fetal-maternal junction, characterized by pleomorphic fetal cells (Krafka, 1941) and necrotic maternal cells. The columns also make contact with each other peripherally to form the cytotrophoblastic shell (fig. 25).

The cytotrophoblastic shell (of Siegenbeek van Heukelom) is the specialized, peripheral part of the cellular trophoblast in contact with maternal tissue. As the shell forms, syncytiotrophoblast is left both internally, where it lines the intervillous space, and externally, where it forms masses that blend with the

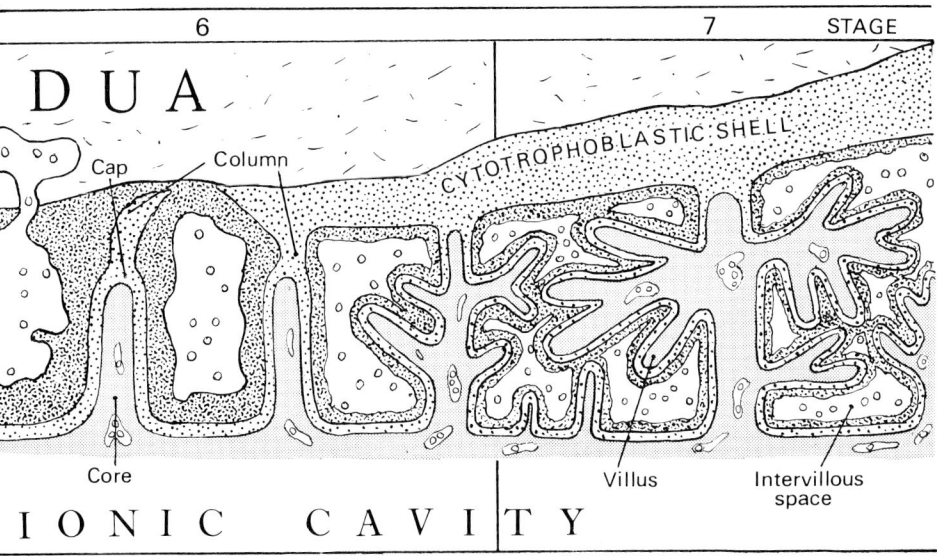

blastic lining for the trophoblast results in a combination known as the chorion. Cytotrophoblastic clumps (stage 5c) acquire mesoblastic crests and become primary villous stems (stage 6). A cytotrophoblastic shell begins to form externally, and free villi project into the intervillous space (stage 7).

decidua. The development and arrangement of the shell have been discussed by Boyd and Hamilton (1970). Defective development of the trophoblast, especially of the shell, results later in villous deficiencies (Grosser, 1926). Moreover, it is important to appreciate that, even in instances where the embryonic disc either fails to form or remains rudimentary, a large chorion with luxuriant villi may still be found.

Because the number of mitotic figures in the cytotrophoblastic covering of a villus is approximately equal to that in the mesoblastic core, Krafka (1941) suggested "that the mesoblast, once established, proliferates at the same rate as the Langhans layer, and hence furnishes its own growth zone." It may be mentioned in passing that the layer featured by Theodor Langhans (in 1870 and subsequently) is the villous cytotrophoblast, "which constitutes the *cellular* (as opposed to *syncytial*) investment of the villi" (Boyd and Hamilton, 1970).

Park (1957) found a low incidence of sex chromatin in the trophoblast and chorionic mesoblast of an embryo (No. 7801) of stage 6, and in the chorionic mesoblast and yolk sac of a second specimen (No. 7762).

Extra-embryonic mesoblast. The chorionic mesoblast is well formed and extends into the villi even in stage 6a, as seen clearly in the Linzenmeier and Peters specimens. Krafka (1941) subscribed to the view (already mentioned) that the chorionic mesoblast arises from the cytotrophoblast, although his agreement seems to have been based largely on the appearance of one cell:

"With the premise that continuity and gradation are not sufficient evidence upon which to establish origin, a search was instituted for a definitely fusiform cell still in unquestionable continuity with the Langhans layer and undergoing mitosis with the cleavage spindle oriented perpendicularly to the Langhans surface. One such cell was found, and three more which fulfilled one but not both requirements. . . . Positive evidence of vasofactive strands was also apparent."

From his acquaintance with Hill's observations of Primates and from his own studies of the Fetzer embryo, Florian (1933) believed in "the existence of an area in the most caudal part of the embryonic disc where the primary mesoderm is fused with the ectoderm." The zone in question may be the site "where primary mesoderm originates (at least in part). This area is situated close behind the primordium of the cloacal membrane" (ibid.), and involves the disc epiblast and the adjoining amniotic ectoderm. This theory of the origin of the primary mesoblast from a localized proliferating area has already been discussed under stage 5c. It should also be pointed out that, in the chick embryo, the caudal half of the primitive streak furnishes only extra-embryonic mesoblast (Nicolet, 1970).

At stage 6a, angiogenesis (see Hertig, 1935) is occurring in the chorionic mesoblast (Nos. 6900 and 6734), blood vessels are found in the villi (No. 6900), and blood islands are seen on the yolk sac (No. 6734). By the end of stage 6b, vascularization of the chorion is almost constant and blood vessels are generally present in the villi (ibid.). Thus, the blood vascular system first arises in extra-embryonic areas. From his studies of chorionic angiogenesis, Hertig (1968) became convinced of "the independent in situ origin of angioblasts and mesoblasts from trophoblast."

Amnion. The amnion is well formed. At its upturned margins, the epiblast of the embryonic disc changes abruptly to the squamous cells of the amnion (fig. 31). Although the amnion appears largely as a single (ectodermal) layer, an external coat of mesoblast can also be detected and, in some places, it "runs along as a layer of mesothelium" (Heuser, Rock, and Hertig, 1945). The amniotic cavity may be either smaller or larger than the yolk sac at stage 6 (fig. 26).

In the Fetzer embryo, among other specimens, Florian (1930a) was able to confirm von Möllendorff's finding in Op of enlargement of the amniotic cavity by epithelial degeneration. An active extension of the amniotic cavity towards the tissue of the connecting stalk took place in a dorsal and caudal direction from the embryonic disc.

The vault of the amniotic cavity may give rise to a diverticulum known as the amniotic duct. The appearances vary from a localized amniotic thickening (in No. 7801) to a pointed process directed towards the trophoblast (in No. 7634, Krafka, 1941, fig. 2, and in No. 7762, Wilson, 1945, fig. 8). The amniotic duct is generally regarded as an inconstant and transitory developmental variation.

Embryonic disc. Terms such as "embryonic disc," "embryonic shield," *Keimscheibe, Embryonalschild,* or "blastodisc" are used in measuring embryos from the rostral amniotic reflexion (Odgers, 1941) to, frequently, the caudal end of the primitive streak (ibid.). Although certain authors (e.g., Grosser, 1931) therefore do not include the cloacal membrane, others (e.g., Florian and Hill, 1935) do include it. When the connecting stalk and allantoic diverticulum are also included, terms such as "embryonic rudiment," *Embryonalanlage, Keimanlage,* or *Keimling* are employed. Many writers do not make clear their points of reference, nor do they always specify whether a measurement has been taken in a straight line (caliper length) or

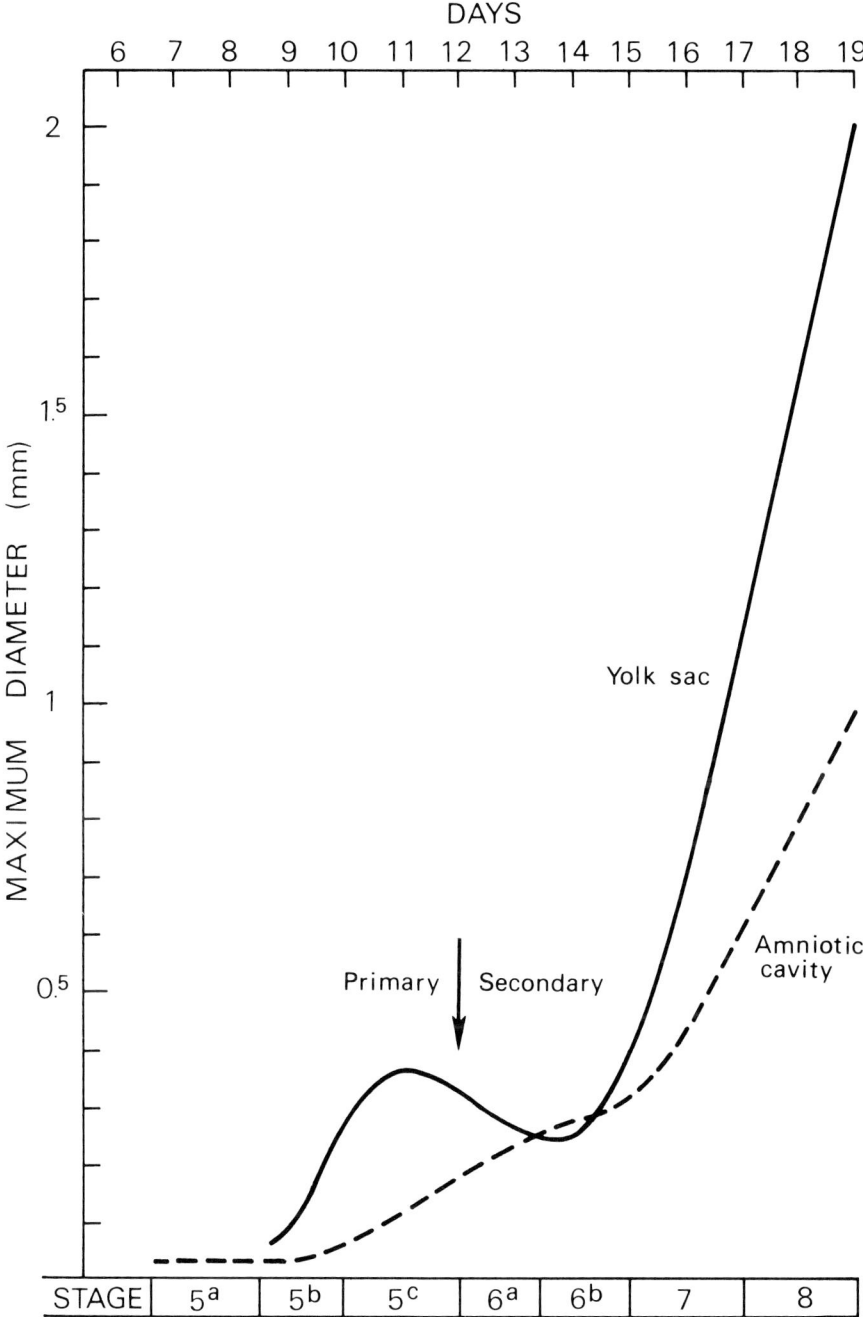

Fig. 26. Graph to show the maximum diameter of the amniotic cavity and of the yolk sac from stages 5 to 8. Based on the measurements of 31 specimens. From stage 5c to stage 6, the primary is transformed into the secondary yolk sac, although the mode of the transformation is not entirely clear. The secondary yolk sac is at first smaller than the primary yolk sac but soon enlarges considerably.

along the curvature of the disc (contour length). In the present work, the "embryonic disc" will be taken to include, where possible, the cloacal membrane, and, except where otherwise specified, the length will generally refer to that measured in a straight line.

As seen from the dorsal aspect, the embryonic disc generally appears elongated, and the long axis of the disc usually (in 10 out of 12 specimens of stage 6b) coincides with that of the primitive streak rather than being at a right angle to it.

Although the dorsal surface of the disc may present some localized convexities and concavities, it is, as a whole, fairly flat. No. 7801, a particularly excellent specimen, is slightly convex (fig. 31) but the marked curvatures illustrated in some embryos (such as T.F.) may be assumed to be artifactual.

A detailed study of the "cytodesmata" in early human embryos was undertaken by Studnička (1929). In two specimens (Bi I and T.F.) of stage 6, cytodesmata were described between the germ layers ("interdermal cytodesmata") and between the mesothelial and the adjacent germ layer in both the amnion and the wall of the yolk sac (Studnička and Florian, 1928).

With the appearance of the primitive streak during stage 6, a process is begun whereby certain cells of the epiblast enter the streak, and the remaining cells on the dorsal aspect of the embryo will become the embryonic ectoderm. The epiblast is continuous with the amniotic ectoderm at the margin of the embryonic disc. The basement membrane (*membrana prima* of Hensen) of the epiblast is clearly visible in a number of stage 6 embryos, such as Harvard No. 55 (where it has been demonstrated histochemically by Hertig et al., 1958), Peters, E.B., Bi I, etc.

The embryonic mesoblast will be discussed under the primitive streak.

The endoderm shows a marked concentration of glycogen, and some of its cells may be primordial germ cells (Hertig et al., 1958). Rostral to the primitive streak, the endoderm consists of large vesicular cells (Heuser, Rock, and Hertig, 1945). It should be kept in mind that, in the chick embryo, it has been shown that the rostral part of the primitive streak (including the node) "always contains a large population of presumptive endoblastic cells" (Nicolet, 1970).

Primitive streak. The primitive streak is a proliferation of cells lying in the median plane in the caudal region of the embryonic disc (figs. 27 and 32). The streak on its first appearance and in narrow usage, is "the thick caudal end of the germ disk" (Heuser and Streeter, 1941). In a much broader and more functional sense, however, "the essential features of the primitive streak are the pluripotential nature of the cells that compose it and the continued segregation of more specialized cells which migrate or delaminate from the less specialized remainder" (*ibid.*).

On the basis of radio-autographic studies of grafts in chick embryos, the primitive streak is believed to be not a blastema but rather "a type of blastopore" in which occur "movement of epiblast toward the streak, invagination at the streak, and subsequent migration to both homolateral and heterolateral mesoderm" (Rosenquist, 1966).[1] Indeed, at primitive streak stages of the chick em-

---

[1] Pasteels (1940) stated that "la thèse faisant de la ligne primitive un blastopore au sens cinétique du mot est défendue" provided it be understood that the blastopore "n'est pas une 'bouche primitive' mais le point d'entreé des cellules à l'intérieur du germe."

bryo, zones have been established for future ectoderm, mesoderm, endoderm, and notochord (*ibid.*). The invagination movements through the primitive streak have been confirmed in xenografts (Vakaet, 1971). Moreover, it is likely that the mammalian pattern is basically similar. In the rabbit, the formation of the embryonic disc and primitive streak "is primarily achieved by migrations of cells that are being rapidly proliferated over the entire surface of the embryonic area. Cell death occurs but is an insignificant factor in this phase of embryonic growth" (Daniel and Olson, 1966).

In the human, the primitive streak appears first during stage 6. The possibility of a streak in some embryos (e.g., Peters) here classified as 6a has been raised. Conversely a streak in at least one 6b embryo (No. 8819) has been denied (Krafka, 1941).

Brewer's (1938) criteria for the presence of a primitive streak are: (1) active proliferation of the cells (shown by a large number of cells in mitosis), (2) the loss of the basement membrane separating the epiblast and endoderm, (3) migration of the epiblastic cells, and (4) intermingling of the cells of the epiblast and endoderm of the disc.

The shape of the early streak is not entirely clear. Brewer (1938) described it as a crescentic formation at the caudal margin of the disc (similar to that seen in the pig) but, as already mentioned, the presence of a streak at all in his specimen, (No. 8819) was denied by Krafka (1941).

In other young 6b embryos (Op, Fetzer, and Wo) the streak possesses the form of a node, and indeed initially "seems to correspond in its position with Hensen's knot" (Florian, 1930a). Thus, in the Fetzer specimen (Fetzer and Florian, 1930), the streak appeared almost circular in dorsal view, was situated not far from the middle of the embryonic disc, and did not reach the cloacal membrane. The question naturally arises as to whether the primordium is not in fact the primitive node rather than the primitive streak in these early specimens. This idea is supported by Dr. J. Jirásek (personal communication, 1970), who believes that the fusion of the epiblast with the endoderm found in this region indicates that the node rather than the streak is involved. According to this interpretation, the primitive node appears during stage 6 and the streak does not appear until the following stage. In the chick embryo, although the streak is said to appear before the node, there is reason to believe that the rostral end of the very young primitive streak already contains the material of the future primitive node (Vakaet, 1960).

When the primitive streak attains a rostrocaudal measurement of 0.1 mm or more, as in Beneke, Am. 10, Bi I, and T.F., its elongation fully justifies the name "streak." By the end of stage 6, both a node and a streak (separated by a "neck") have been recorded in one (somewhat abnormal) embryo (HEB-18, Mazanec, 1960).

In the first specimens of stage 6b (Liverpool I and II, No. 7801, No. 8819, No. 7762, Op, Fetzer), the length of the primitive streak is less than one quarter that of the embryonic disc. In Wo and Beneke it is less than one third, and in Am. 10, Bi I, and T.F. it is less than one half. Finally, in the transitional and somewhat abnormal HEB-18 specimen, the streak attains one half the length of the embryonic disc.

The primitive groove appears probably during stage 6b. At any rate its presence has been claimed in some specimens

(Liverpool II, Op, and T.F.) of that stage (fig. 32).

Although it may be possible at least in some instances, to ascertain the rostro-caudal axis of the embryo at stages 5c and 6a, unequivocal manifestation awaits the initial appearance of the primitive streak during stage 6b (O'Rahilly, 1970). With the establishment of bilateral symmetry, the embryonic disc, in addition to its dorsal and ventral surfaces, now has rostral and caudal ends and right and left sides. The median plane[2] may be defined, and the terms "medial" and "lateral" are applicable. Moreover, it is proper to speak of coronal (or frontal), sagittal, and transverse planes. The last-named, in anticipation of the erect posture, may be termed horizontal. Certain other terms, however, such as "anterior," "posterior," "superior," and "inferior," should be avoided at this period because of their special meaning in adult human anatomy.

Embryonic mesoblast. At first, the embryonic mesoblast is scarcely recognizable as such (Nos. 8819 and 7762) or is quite scanty in amount (No. 7801). Although the main bulk of the embryonic mesoblast is believed to come by way of the primitive streak, other sources are not excluded. Lateral to the streak, for example, it is possible that some epiblastic cells bypass the streak and migrate locally into the mesoblast (Heuser, Rock, and Hertig, 1945). In addition, the possibility of contributions from the gut endoderm has been raised in the case of the macaque (Heuser and Streeter, 1941). Finally, the degree of incorporation of some of the primary mesoblast

[2] The terms "median sagittal" and "parasagittal" are redundant. The median plane is sagittal by definition and anything parallel with a sagittal plane is still sagittal. This usage has been accepted in all the recognized anatomical terminologies.

into definitive body mesoderm is unknown. Conversely, in the Beneke specimen, Florian (1933) "could trace the secondary mesoderm behind the caudal end of the primitive streak around the cloacal membrane into the connecting stalk." (The very closely arranged cells of the secondary mesoblast were distinguishable from the looser cells of the primary tissue.) Hence, the convenient distinction between primary and secondary mesoblast should not be interpreted too rigidly. A need exists for further detailed studies of the distribution and spread of mesoblast during these early stages.

In the chick embryo, at the stage of the definitive streak, it has been "established that each [topographical] kind of mesoblast has a definite place along the cephalo-caudal axis of the primitive streak, precise enough to be demonstrated experimentally" (Nicolet, 1970).

Prechordal plate. The earliest human embryo in which the prechordal plate has been recorded seems to be Beneke at stage 6b. In that specimen, "in front of, and below the cranial extremity of the primitive streak . . . the endoderm is distinctly thickened and proliferative" in "a horseshoe shaped area;" that area "must be regarded as a mesoderm producing zone" (Hill and Florian, 1963). Study of later specimens, such as Manchester 1285 and Dobbin, led Hill and Florian to "regard the thickened area in question as prechordal plate." Dr. W. P. Luckett has called the writer's attention to several stage 5c specimens (Nos. 7950, 8558, and 8330) in which the endoderm appears to be thickened at one end of the embryo, as shown in the photomicrographs published by Hertig, Rock, and Adams (1956, figs. 35, 37, and 38).

It is of interest to note that, in *Tarsius*, the prechordal plate, which later adopts the form of an annular zone, is at first represented by a continuous sheet of thickened endoderm underlying most of the embryonic epiblast (Hill and Florian, 1963).

Yolk sac (fig. 31). The yolk sac functions "as a specialized nutritional membrane" (Streeter, 1937) and, in addition, serves as the site of origin of primordial germ cells as well as an important temporary locus of hematopoietic activity (Hoyes, 1969).

From stage 5c to stage 6, the primary is transformed into the secondary yolk sac (fig. 26), although the mode of the transformation has long been disputed. (See Stieve, 1931; Heuser and Streeter, 1941; Strauss, 1945; Hamilton and Boyd, 1950; Starck, 1956.)

According to Hertig (1968), the primary yolk sac "blows up" or "pops," and the torn edges that remain attached to the endoderm coalesce to form the secondary yolk sac. The secondary sac "soon takes on a second or inner layer of epithelial nature" (*ibid.*) which is, in Hertig's view, derived from the wall of the yolk sac itself. In other words, "endodermal" cells differentiate *in situ* from the mesothelium of the exocoelomic membrane (Streeter, 1937).

According to a number of other authors (such as Stieve, 1931), however, "it seems likely that endoderm from the edge of the embryonic disc proliferates and migrates round the interior" of the exocoelomic membrane (Hamilton and Boyd, 1950), using that membrane "as a guiding surface" (Mazanec, 1953).

A further possibility is the dehiscence of cells from the disc endoderm so that a new cavity is formed between the two endodermal layers or possibly between the disc endoderm and the dorsal part of the exocoelomic membrane.

In any case, it appears likely that, at least in some embryos, the distal part of the primary yolk sac becomes detached from the proximal part, thereby forming one or more isolated vesicles or cysts (see below). As a result of these processes, the secondary yolk sac is at first smaller than the primary yolk sac (fig. 26).

The external and internal strata of the now bilaminar yolk sac are commonly referred to as the mesodermal and endodermal layers, respectively. Three layers can be distinguished later on (e.g., by stage 10): mesothelium, mesenchyme, and endodermal epithelium (Hesseldahl and Larsen, 1969).

In a number of embryos of stage 6 (such as No. 7634) and some subsequent stages, a diverticulum of the yolk sac has been recorded. These outgrowths arise generally at the abembryonic pole of the yolk sac. They vary from slight evaginations to long processes (0.45 mm in Liverpool II, for example), and are frequently associated with cysts. It has been suggested that the diverticula and cysts are remnants of the primary yolk sac (Heuser, Rock, and Hertig, 1945).

Cloacal membrane. The cloacal membrane appears during stage 6b. Although at least its site may be detected in the first specimens of that stage (such as No. 7801), the membrane is probably present in all specimens that possess a primitive streak of 0.05 mm or more in length. The membrane is at first a cell cord that connects the epiblast with the endoderm (Florian, 1933) and is of variable length (about 0.015 to 0.025 mm). Later (stage 7) it increases in size and begins to assume the form of an actual membrane.

Allantoic diverticulum. The existence of an allantois in the human remained controversial until the end of the nineteenth century (Meyer, 1953). In early embryos, the recognition of an allantoic primordium presents considerable difficulty. A recess of the yolk sac, such as appears in embryo Op, should not be assumed to be necessarily the allantois. According to Florian (1930), "the yolk-sac penetrates into the connecting stalk in the form of a narrow diverticulum which enlarges and eventually opens out again into the cavity of the yolk sac. This process may probably be repeated several times." Hence some reservations must be made concerning the "allanto-enteric diverticulum" of Liverpool I. In No. 7801, all that is found is merely "a tiny recess in the wall of the yolk sac at the spot where the allantoic duct presumably originates" (Heuser, Rock, and Hertig, 1945). In Wo, a solid *Allantois-anlage* has been claimed. In Beneke, the yolk sac diverticulum is not the allantois (Florian and Beneke, 1931). In Bi I, the appearance of the diverticulum has been attributed to "a ventral down-bulging of the underlying wall of the yolk-sac" produced by the end node of the primitive streak (Florian, 1930a). The condition in T.F. may well be similar. In conclusion, it is difficult to find a convincing example of an allanto-enteric diverticulum at stage 6.

Connecting stalk. Florian (1930) pointed out that the connecting stalk (as exemplified in embryo Op) comprises two portions (fig. 27): (a) the amnio-embryonic stalk, an attachment of the entire amnio-embryonic vesicle to the chorionic mesoderm, and (b) the umbilical stalk, by which the caudal end of the embryo is anchored to the chorion. The umbilical stalk, which is in all stages covered on its cranial surface by amniotic ectoderm, later becomes transformed into the umbilical cord.

The Peters embryo is situated in a thickening of the chorionic mesoderm but the connecting stalk is "not yet present" (Florian, 1930a). Although "a body stalk proper has not yet fully formed" in No. 7634 (Krafka, 1941), its primordium is present and comprises the amnio-embryonic and umbilical stalks of Florian. The condition is similar to that in Op, in which Florian has pointed out that the axis of the connecting stalk has already begun to form an acute angle (open caudally) with the embryonic plate. By the end of stage 6b, blood vessel primordia are present in the developing stalk and indicate the future umbilical vessels (Hertig, 1935). In the opinion of Hill and Florian (1963), the vessels of the connecting stalk in *Tarsius* "can arise directly as invaginations of the mesothelium" covering the stalk.

SPECIMENS OF STAGE 6 IN CARNEGIE COLLECTION

These are listed in order of serial number in Table 12. Because not all of these embryos have been investigated specifically for the presence of axial features, a distinction between 6a and 6b will not be made in the Table.

SPECIMENS OF STAGE 6a ALREADY DESCRIBED

Carnegie No. 8905, Merrill. Unbranched villi. Although an abnormal leucocytic reaction is present, this specimen "represents the best example in the author's collection of formation of early primordial villi, active mesogenesis and angiogenesis, completion of the amnion and the transitional phase between the primary and definitive [secondary] yolk sac formation" (Hertig, 1968, who reproduced a photomicrograph as fig. 55). Presumed age, 12–13 days.

Carnegie No. 6800, Stöckel. Described by Linzenmeier (1914). Hysterectomy.

STAGE 6

TABLE 12. List of Specimens of Stage 6 in Carnegie Collection

Serial No.	Grade	Fixative	Cutting Medium	Thinness (micrometers)	Stain	Date and Donor	Remarks and Reference
6026	Poor	?	?	6?	H.-E.	1929, C. Lockyer, London	Lockyer embryo. Abnormal. Ramsey, 1937
6734	Poor	Zenker-acetic	P	10	H.-E.	1934, R. Hussey, New Haven, Conn.	Yale embryo. Ramsey, 1938
6900	Poor	Formal.	P	15	H.-E.	1940, R. Meyer, Berlin	Linzenmeier, 1914
7634	Poor	Formal.	P	10	H.-E. etc.	1940, J. Krafka, Augusta, Ga.	Torpin embryo. Krafka, 1941
7762	Good	Zenker-formal.	P	8	?	1940, K. M. Wilson, Rochester, N.Y.	Wilson, 1945
7800	Exc.	?	C-P	8	H.-E.	1940, J. Rock & A. T. Hertig, Boston, Mass.	Abnormal
7801	Exc.	Bouin	C-P	8	H.-E.	1940, A. T. Hertig, Boston, Mass.	Heuser et al., 1945
7850	Exc.	Alc. & Bouin	C-P	6	H.-E.	1940, A. T. Hertig, Boston, Mass.	Abnormal
8290	Exc.	Bouin	C-P	8	H.-phlox.	1944, A. T. Hertig, Boston, Mass.	
8360	Exc.	Alc. & Bouin	C-P	6	H.-E. phlox.	1944, A. T. Hertig, Boston, Mass.	
8362	Poor	?	C-P	6	H.-E. phlox.	1944, A. T. Hertig, Boston, Mass.	
8672	Exc.	Alc. & Bouin	C-P	6	H.-E.	1949, A. T. Hertig, Boston, Mass.	
8819	Exc.	Formal.-chrom. subl.	C-P	8	H.-E.	1951, J. I. Brewer, Chicago, Ill.	Edwards-Jones-Brewer (H.1496). Brewer, 1938
8905	Poor	Alc.	P	6	H.-E. phlox.	1951, A. T. Hertig, Boston, Mass.	Abnormal
8910	Good	Formal.	C-P	8	H.-E. phlox.	1951, C. H. Heuser, Augusta, Ga.	
9222	Good	Bouin	C-P	6 & 10	Azan	1954, R. E. Johnstone, Cincinnati, Ohio	Abnormal. Possibly stage 7
9250	Exc.	Bouin	P	8	H.-E.	1954, A. T. Hertig, Boston, Mass.	
9595	Poor	?	P	8	H.-E.	1958, City of Baltimore	
10003	Good	Bouin	P	5	Various	1963, W. S. Hammond, Syracuse, N.Y.	

Angiogenesis in chorion described by Hertig (1935). Photomicrographs reproduced by Hertig (1968, figs. 56–58). Important as one of the youngest specimens having "true villi" (Hertig and Rock, 1941). Chorionic villi show "an occasional tendency to dichotomous branching" (Krafka, 1941). Indication of blood vessel formation in villi. Chorion, 2.75 × 1.05 × 0.9 mm. Chorionic cavity, 0.75 × 0.61 × 0.52 mm; capacity, 0.13 mm^3 (Odgers, 1937). Embryonic disc, 0.21 × 0.105 mm (Krafka, 1941). Allantoic diverticulum doubtful. Presumed age, 13 days (*ibid.*).

Carnegie No. 8672. Photomicrograph illustrated by Hertig, Rock, and Adams (1956, fig. 40). Chorion, 1.14 × 1.08 mm. Chorionic cavity, 0.8 × 0.79 mm. Embryonic disc, 0.203 × 0.07 mm. Presumed age, 13 days.

Harvard No. 55. Studied histochemically by Hertig *et al.* (1958). Hysterectomy. Chorion, 1.77 × 1.33 × 0.598 mm. Chorionic cavity, 0.73 × 0.68 × 0.221 mm. Embryonic disc, 0.296 × 0.196 × 0.044 mm. Chorionic villi essentially solid, with earliest suggestion of mesoblastic core formation. "Apparently without axial differentiation." Possesses "a very recently formed definitive [secondary] yolk sac." Possible primordial germ cells ("stuffed with glycogen") within endoderm near edge of disc. Presumed age, 13 days. For histochemical details, the original paper should be consulted.

Carnegie No. 8360. Photomicrographs illustrated by Hertig, Rock, and Adams (1956, figs. 42 and 46). Chorion, 1.466 × 1 mm. Chorionic cavity, 1 × 0.66 mm. Embryonic disc, 0.188 × 0.055 mm. Presumed age, 13 days.

Peters. Described in a monograph by Peters (1899). Autopsy. A famous embryo, for long the youngest known and the first to be described in detail. Photomicrographs have since been published (Rossenbeck, 1923, plate 42; Odgers, 1937, plate 2, fig. 2). The chorionic villi, some of which display a mesenchymal core, send cellular columns externally and these latter are beginning to form a cytotrophoblastic shell. Slight branching of villi (Krafka, 1941). Chorionic cavity contains magma réticulé of Velpeau (Mall, 1916). Blood islands on yolk sac. Chorion, 1.5 × 2 mm. Chorionic cavity, 1.6 × 0.9 × 0.8 mm; capacity, 0.7 mm^3 (Odgers, 1937). Embryonic disc, 0.18 × 0.24 mm (Krafka, 1941). The basement membrane (Hensen's *membrana prima*) of the epiblast was noted by Graf Spee. Allantoic diverticulum and primitive streak uncertain. Presumed age, 13 days (Krafka, 1941). A tabulation of normal human embryos compiled from the literature prior to 1900 and from Mall's own collection was published by Mall (1900, pp. 38–46). The least advanced specimen was the Peters embryo, and included in the list were 92 embryos from 0.19 to 32 mm, as well as 17 fetuses from 33 to 210 mm.

E.B. (E. Béla v. Entz). Described by Faber (1940). Curettage. Incomplete. Primitive villi. Chorionic cavity, 0.935 × 0.697 mm. Embryonic disc, 0.231 mm. No primitive streak, node, or groove. Secondary yolk sac. No allantoic diverticulum. Said to resemble the Peters specimen closely.

Carnegie No. 7634, Torpin. Described in detail by Krafka (1941), who provided also an extensive discussion of the decidua. Hysterectomy. Posterior wall of uterus. Chorionic villi with mesoblastic cores, 0.1–0.2 mm in length. Villi "generally single, but two or more may arise from a common base," although no branching was recorded. Chorion (possessed 85 villi), 1.76 × 1.7 × 1.5 mm. Chorionic cavity, 1.3 × 1.1 × 1 mm. Embryonic disc, 0.216 × 0.21 mm. Amniotic duct. Neither primitive node nor primitive streak. Cloacal cord (rather than membrane) claimed, but doubted by Mazanec (1959). No allantoic diverticulum. Yolk sac diverticulum. Presumed age, 13 days. Dorsal and transverse projections published (Krafka, 1941, figs. 1 and 3, and plate 2).

VMA-1. Specimen of Knorre, summarized by Mazanec (1959). Chorion, 3.24 × 2.04 mm. Chorionic cavity, 1.53 × 1.02 mm. Embryonic disc, 0.23 × 0.2 mm. Development thought to be between Torpin and Yale specimens.

Carnegie No. 6734, Yale. Described in detail by Ramsey (1938). Necropsy. Left lateral uterine wall. Chorion, 2.75 × 1.9 × 0.76 mm. Chorionic cavity, 1.3 × 1.1 × 1 mm. Some of the chorionic villi "show dichotomous division, but no more complicated branching has occurred." Some angioblastic strands in villi. Embryonic disc (damaged and distorted), 0.15 mm. Allantoic diverticulum stated to be present but denied by Krafka (1941). Presumed age, 13–14 days. Drawings of model published (Ramsey, 1938, fig. 1).

An autopsy specimen described by Noback, Paff, and Poppiti (1968) possessed a chorion of 2.25 × 1.25 × 2 mm. Chorionic villi avascular. Embryonic disc, 0.22 × 0.2 mm. No primitive node, notochordal process, cloacal membrane, or allantoic diverticulum. Axial differentiation, however, was suggested by the possible primordia of the prechordal plate and the primitive streak. Hence this specimen may be regarded as transitional between 6a and 6b.

SPECIMENS OF STAGE 6b ALREADY DESCRIBED

(listed in order of length of primitive streak)

Liverpool I. Described by Harrison and Jeffcoate (1953). Curettage. Chorionic villi "are only beginning to show evidence of branching (*ibid.*, Plate 1, fig. 1)." Chorion, 1.86 × 1.47 mm. Chorionic cavity, 1.5 × 0.84 mm. Embryonic disc, 0.161 × 0.199 × 0.033 mm. Primitive streak, 0.021 mm. Allanto-enteric diverticulum claimed. Median projection published (*ibid.*, fig. 1; Mazanec, 1959, fig. 31).

Liverpool II. Described by Lewis and Harrison (1966), who, in view of "the dimensions, degree of differentiation and decidual appearances," assigned the specimen to horizon VII. Hysterectomy. The chorionic villi are localized to the embryonic pole, and their mesoblastic cores contain "isolated vascular primordia formed by coalescence of angioblasts." "The villi are branched; lacunae and intervillous spaces have formed." Chorion, 2.72 × 2.35 × 1.54 mm. Embryonic disc, 0.264 × 0.22 mm. Primitive streak, 0.024 mm. Amniotic duct and long yolk sac duct. Resembles Teacher-Bryce II embryo. Median projection published (*ibid.*, fig. 6).

Carnegie No. 7801 (figs. 27–32). Described in detail and illustrated by Heuser, Rock, and Hertig (1945). Hysterectomy. Posterior wall of uterus. "The primitive villi are short and stubby; a few reach a length of about 0.25 mm." Chorion, 2.6 × 1.9 × 1.4 mm. Chorionic cavity, 1.3 × 1.1 × 0.8 mm. Embryonic disc, 0.04 × 0.22 × 0.253 mm. Primitive streak, 0.04 mm. "Axial differentiation is just appearing." "In this embryo the site of the future [cloacal] membrane seems indicated, but not the structure

Fig. 27. Dorsal view and median reconstruction of No. 7801, stage 6, in alignment. The dorsal view, which is based on a graphic reconstruction by the present writer, shows the location of the primitive streak and primitive groove. The median reconstruction is based on a drawing by Mr. Didusch (Heuser, Rock, and Hertig, 1945, Plate 3). The primitive streak is indicated by vertical lines, and the cross-hatched area (containing a mark of interrogation) suggests the site of the future cloacal membrane. The system of shading is further clarified in figure 33. The connecting stalk comprises amnio-embryonic and umbilical stalks. The figure references are to the sections reproduced by Heuser, Rock, and Hertig (1945, Plates 1 and 2).

STAGE 6

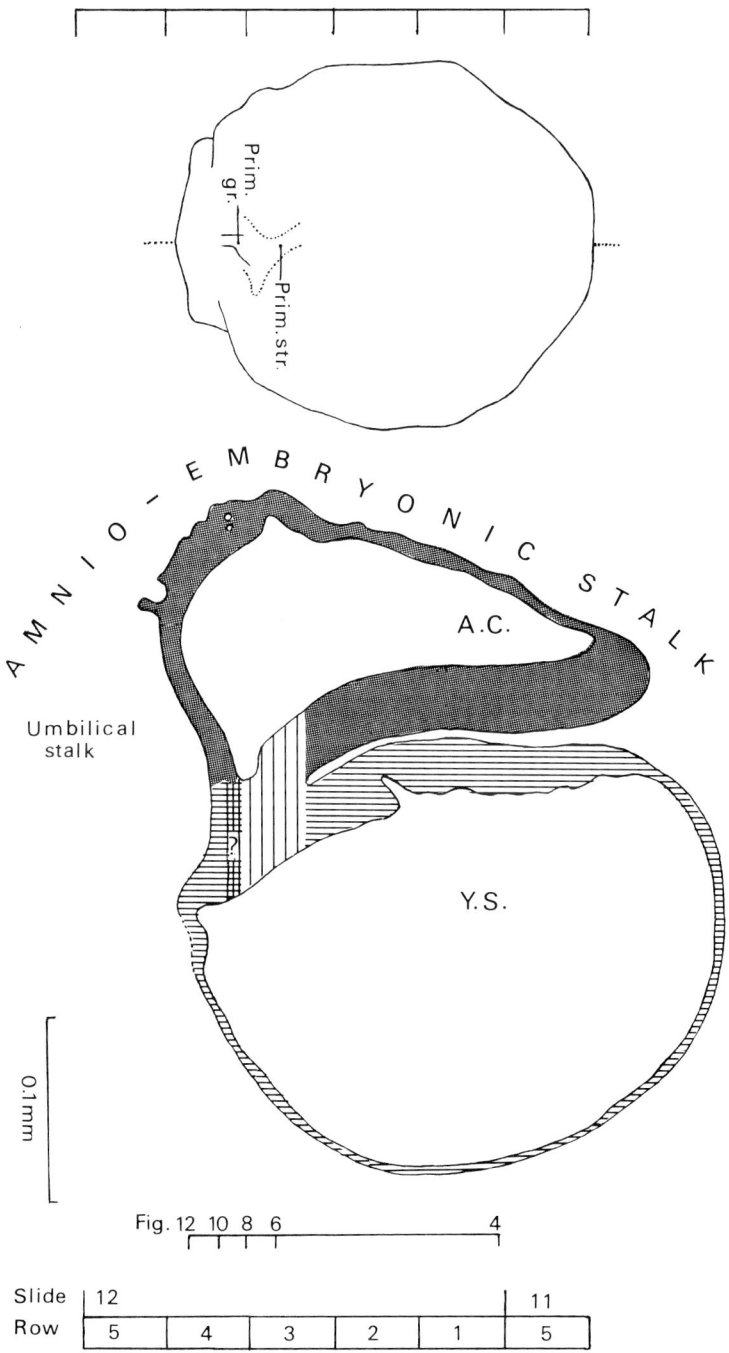

Fig. 28. Surface view of the implantation site of No. 7801, stage 6. A small amount of maternal blood escaped and coagulated on one side of the elevated area.

Fig. 29. Side view of the implantation site of No. 7801, stage 6.

Fig. 30. General view of the tissues at and near the implantation site (No. 7801, stage 6) to show the scab (*Schlusscoagulum*) of hemorrhagic exudate, actual hemorrhage underlying the scab, primary villous stems, blood-filled uterine glands, and early decidua. The embryo is evident, and, near the opposite wall of the chorion, a vesicle presumed to be a detached part of the yolk sac can be identified. Section 12-1-1.

STAGE 6

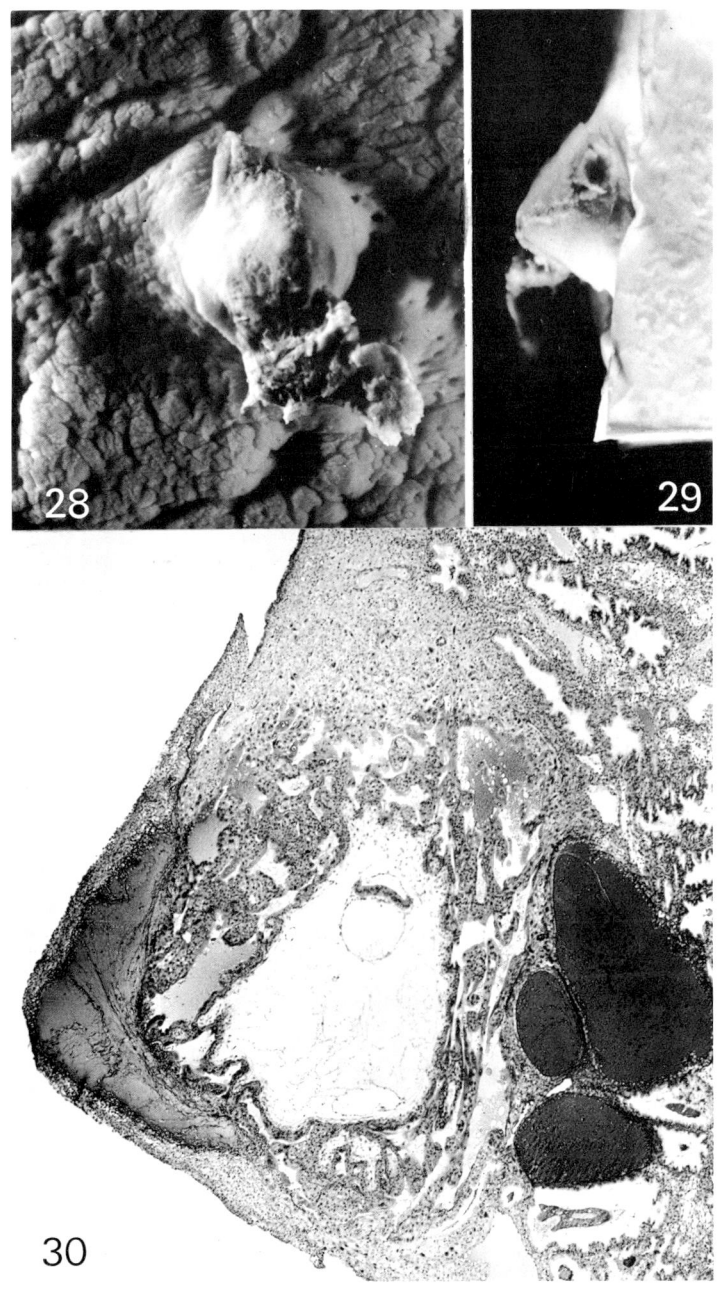

Fig. 31. The amniotic cavity, embryonic disc, and yolk sac of No. 7801, stage 6. The upturned margins of the epiblast change abruptly to the squamous cells of the amniotic ectoderm. The gut endoderm has a foamy appearance, whereas the cells lining the yolk sac are squamous. The yolk sac has acquired an external coat. Section 12-1-1.

Fig. 32. The embryonic disc of No. 7801, stage 6, in the region of the primitive streak. The connecting stalk, the amniotic cavity, and the yolk sac are also visible. Section 12-3-6.

STAGE 6

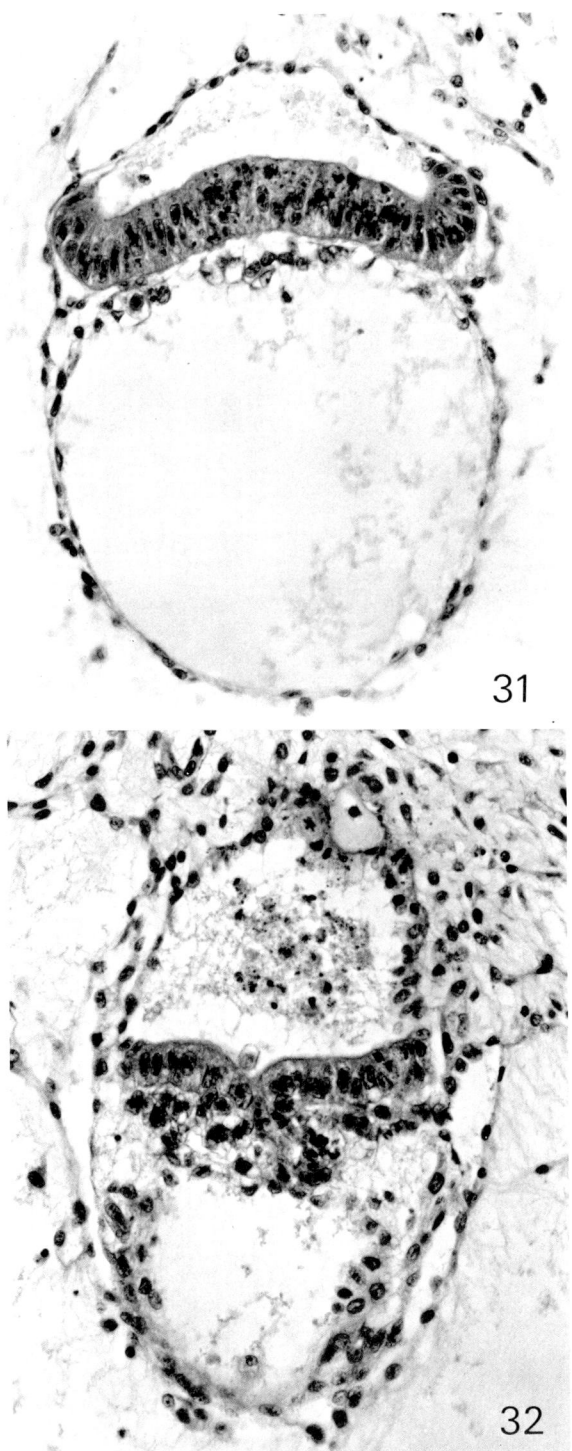

itself." Probably no allantoic duct. Presumed age, 13 or 13½ days. Median projection published (*ibid.*, plate 3).

Carnegie No. 8819, Edwards-Jones-Brewer. Described in detail by Brewer (1937, 1938). Hysterectomy. "There is no branching of a mesodermal villus." Chorion, 3.6 × 3 × 1.9 mm. Chorionic cavity, 1.85 × 1.71 × 1.01 mm; capacity, 13.38 mm³. Embryonic disc, 0.209 × 0.177 mm; volume, 0.0814 mm³. Primitive streak, 0.04 mm, claimed, but its presence was denied by Krafka (1941). No allantoic diverticulum. Dorsal and median projections published (Brewer, 1938, plate 1, figs. 2 and 3; Mazanec, 1959, fig. 33). Some authors have attempted to identify a prechordal plate from the median projection.

Carnegie No. 7762, Rochester. Described by Wilson (1945). Curettage. Chorion, 2.3 × 2.2 × 2 mm. Larger villi have a mesoblastic core "and some show a tendency toward branching." Moreover, "no evidence of actual blood vessels is seen in the villi, but in many of them . . . groupings of angioblasts . . . are observed." Chorionic cavity, 1.75 × 1.3 × 1 mm. Embryonic disc, 0.313 × 0.22 mm. Primitive streak, 0.04 mm. No definite allantoic diverticulum. Amniotic duct. Median reconstruction published (*ibid.*, plate 3; Mazanec, 1959, fig. 36).

Op (Opitz). Described by von Möllendorff (1921b). Hysterectomy. Chorionic villi show first branching in many places. Chorionic cavity, 1.5 × 1.15 × 1 mm. Embryonic disc, 0.19 mm. Primitive streak, 0.045 mm. Allantoic diverticulum denied by Florian (1930). Disintegrating epithelial proliferation of amnion behind caudal end of embryonic plate (Florian, 1930). Median reconstruction published (Mazanec, 1959, fig. 34).

Fetzer. Described by Fetzer (1910) and by Fetzer and Florian (1929, 1930).

Curettage. Chorionic villi "show a beginning tendency to branch" (Streeter, 1920). Chorion, 2.2 × 1.8 mm. Chorionic cavity, 1.6 × 0.9 mm. Embryonic disc, 0.26 × 0.215 mm. Primitive streak (denied by Rossenbeck, 1923), 0.05 mm. Cloacal membrane (Florian, 1933) but no allantoic diverticulum. Area of mesoblastic proliferation from adjacent disc and amniotic ectoderm, "caudal" to cloacal membrane (Hill, 1932; Florian, 1933). Stated to lie between Wo and Bi I in development. Dorsal and median projections published (Fetzer and Florian, 1930, figs. 1a, 1b, 2, and 53; Florian, 1946, plate 4, fig. 40; Mazanec, 1959, fig. 37).

H.R. 1 (Hesketh Roberts). Described by Johnston (1940), who included Florian's divergent interpretation of the specimen. Hysterectomy. Chorion and endometrium described by Johnston (1941). According to Florian, the embryonic disc is 0.048 mm and the primitive streak is 0.06 mm in length. Primitive node, notochordal process, and prechordal plate all absent (but described as present by Johnston). Embryo abnormal in shape, the result of an abnormal growth process. Median projection published (Johnston, 1940, fig. 35).

Wo (Wolfring). Described by von Möllendorff (1925). Chorionic cavity, 2.52 × 2.16 × 2.06 mm. Embryonic disc, 0.25 × 0.22 mm. Primitive streak, 0.065 mm. Cloacal membrane rather than solid allantois (Florian, 1933). Median projection published (von Möllendorff, 1925, fig. 4; Florian, 1928, fig. 40; Mazanec, 1959, fig. 38).

Beneke (Strahl-Beneke). Described originally by Strahl and Beneke in 1916 in a monograph and later by Florian and Beneke (1931). Chorionic cavity, 3.8 × 2.2 × 1.2 mm. Embryonic disc (narrow type), 0.375 mm (Florian,

1934). Primitive streak (doubted by Rossenbeck, 1923, and denied by Fahrenholz, 1927, but acknowledged by Florian, 1928), 0.1 mm. No notochordal process (Hill and Florian, 1931b). Prechordal plate 0.066 mm. Dorsal and median projections published (Florian and Beneke, 1931, figs. 2 and 1; Florian, 1928, fig. 42; Florian, 1946, plate 4, fig. 41; Mazanec, 1959, fig. 40).

Am. 10. Described by Krause (1953). Hysterectomy. Chorionic cavity, 3.6 × 2.5 × 2.5 mm. Embryonic disc (broad type), 0.32 × 0.3 × 0.06 mm. Primitive streak, 0.135 mm. No notochordal process (but see Mazanec, 1959) although a small lumen was suggested as a possible Anlage of "Lieberkühn's canal." Dorsal and median projections published (Krause, 1953, figs. 13 and 15; Mazanec, 1959, fig. 42).

Bi I (Bittman). Described by Florian (1927) and in 1928 in a Czech publication. (For general appearance, see Mazanec, 1959, figs. 95 and 112.) Chorionic cavity, 2.13 × 2.13 × 2.12 mm. Embryonic disc (broad type), 0.35 × 0.34 mm. Primitive streak, which appears as an "indifferent cellular knot" (Florian, 1928), 0.135 mm. Possible primordial germ cell in ventral wall of yolk sac (Politzer, 1933). Median projection published (Florian, 1928, fig. 41; Florian, 1946, plate 5, fig. 42; Mazanec, 1959, fig. 41).

Lbg (Lönnberg). Described by Holmdahl (1939). Chorion, 16 × 15 mm. Embryonic disc, 0.285 × 0.236 × 0.032 mm. Primitive streak, 0.144 mm. No allantoic duct.

T.F. Described by Florian (1927, 1928). Autopsy. Chorionic cavity, 4.578 × 3.078 × 1.76 mm. Embryonic disc, 0.468 × 0.397 × 0.485 mm. Primitive streak (Mazanec, 1959, fig. 100), 0.162 mm. No notochordal process.

Median projection published (Florian, 1928, figs. 27 and 43; Mazanec, 1959, fig. 43).

HEB-18. Described by Mazanec (1960). Abortion. Abnormal features. Chorionic cavity, 4.29 × 4 × 3.55 mm. Embryonic disc (broad type), 0.44 × 0.47 mm. Primitive streak, 0.187–0.22 mm, and node, 0.071 mm. No notochordal process. Dorsal and median projections published (*ibid.*, figs. 1 and 2). Regarded as transitional between stages 6 and 7.

ADDITIONAL SPECIMENS

In the case of the following embryos, a precise measurement of the primitive streak has not been provided in the accounts of the specimens. They are listed in order of year of publication.

Minot. Described by Lewis in Keibel and Mall (1912). Primitive streak present. Median projection published (*ibid.*, vol. 2, fig. 229).

An autopsy specimen described by Schlagenhaufer and Verocay (1916) possessed an embryonic disc of 0.24 × 0.28 mm. Although a primitive streak was not found, the development of the specimen is such that it was probably present (Mazanec, 1959).

Teacher-Bryce II. Described by Bryce (1924) and M'Intyre (1926). Autopsy. Chorionic villi are "well developed but are still simple and little branched." Chorion, 4.5 × 4 × 3.5 mm. Chorionic cavity, 2.8 × 2.6 × 2.25 mm. Embryonic disc, 0.2 × 0.1 × 0.15 mm. Primitive streak present (Mazanec, 1959). Long yolk sac stalk. Blood vessel primordia in connecting stalk.

H 381. Described by Stump (1929). Chorionic villi branched. Chorion, 4.38 × 4.2 × 1.4 mm. Chorionic cavity, 3.48 × 3.44 × 0.81 mm. Embryonic disc, 0.58 × 0.3 mm. Primitive groove and streak or node believed to be present. Said to resemble Hugo and Debeyre specimens.

Andô. Described by Hiramatsu (1936). Hysterectomy. Chorion, 4.2 × 3.25 × 1.9 mm. Chorionic cavity, 4.2 × 2.4 × 1 mm. Embryonic disc, 0.24 × 0.26 × 0.04 mm. Some villi branched. Stated to resemble the Peters specimen. Described as possessing no primitive streak but Mazanec (1959) detected a very early Anlage of the primitive streak in one of the illustrations. Presumed age, 14–15 days. A median interpretation has been published (Mazanec, 1959, fig. 35).

Carnegie No. 6026, Lockyer. A pathological specimen described by Ramsey (1937). Necropsy. Branching villi. Chorionic cavity, 2.12 × 1.48 × 1.6 mm. Embryonic disc degenerated. Primitive groove and embryonic mesoblast probably present. Formerly classified under horizon VIII.

Thomson. Described by Odgers (1937). Chorionic cavity, 2.1 × 1.51 × 0.7 mm; capacity, 1.55 mm.³ Embryonic disc (which shows "a good deal of disorganization"), 0.26 × 0.31 (?) × 0.16 (?) mm. Compared by author to various stage 6 embryos.

Fife-Richter. Described briefly in an abstract by Richter (1952). Hysterectomy. Branching villi. Chorion, 3.44 mm. Chorionic cavity, 2.24 mm. Embryonic disc, 0.29 × 0.4 mm. "A poorly defined primitive streak with groove is present."

A specimen described by Kistner (1953) included only one slide through the embryonic disc. Curettage. Primitive streak thought to be present. Presumed age, 13 days.

A specimen described by Jahnke and Stegner (1964) possessed a chorionic cavity of 2.5 × 2.3 × 1.5 mm. Embryonic disc, 0.31 × 0.29 mm. Primitive streak not precisely ascertainable but thought to be present. Presumed age, 15–16 days. Median projection published (*ibid.*, fig. 2).

Twins have been described by Hamilton, Boyd, and Misch (1967). Hysterectomy. Chorion 2.37 × 2 × 1.4 mm. Early villi. Embryonic disc with primitive node. Twin represented by (1) a vesicle interpreted as "a poorly developed embryonic disc and amnion," and (2) a detached yolk sac. Monozygotic twinning here due probably to unequal division of inner cell mass of blastocyst.

Carnegie No. 8290. Abnormal specimen illustrated by Hertig (1968, fig. 129). Polypoid implantation site, deficient polar trophoblast, and buckled embryonic disc. Presumed age, 13 days.

Carnegie No. 7800. Abnormal specimen illustrated by Hertig (1968, fig. 126). Trophoblastic hypoplasia with virtual absence of chorionic villi. Presumed age, 13 days. Thought to belong to either stage 6 or stage 7.

Several other unsatisfactory specimens (in poor condition or inadequately described or both) have been published but will not be referred to here. These include Bayer (Keibel, 1890) and von Herff (v. Spee, 1896), and the specimens of Giacomini (1898), van Heukelom (1898), Jung (1908), Herzog (1909), Heine and Hofbauer (1911), Johnstone (1914), Greenhill (1927), and Thomas and van Campenhout (1953). These probably belong to stage 6 and further examples may be found in Mazanec (1959). Moreover, frankly pathological specimens have also been recorded, e.g., by Harrison, Jones, and Jones (1966).

STAGE 7

Stage 7 is characterized by the appearance of the notochordal process (figs. 33 and 36). The maximum diameter of the chorion varies from 4 to 9 mm, that of the chorionic cavity from 1.5 to 8 mm. The embryonic disc is generally 0.3 to 0.7 mm in length but varies from 0.1 to 1 mm. The age is believed to be about 16 days.

In Streeter's (1942) scheme, horizon VII was characterized by "branching villi, axis of germ disk defined." Such specimens are here classified in stage 6b because (1) some branching of villi has been recorded even in certain stage 6a (horizon VI) embryos (e.g., No. 6734: "occasionally they [the villi] show dichotomous division . . .," Ramsey, 1938), and is of scant use, therefore, as a criterion; (2) the embryonic axis is defined in some embryos already admitted to horizon VI (e.g., No. 7801, which shows "the primordium of the primitive streak," Hertig, Rock, and Adams, 1956). Moreover, embryos already assigned to horizon VII (e.g., No. 7802) show additional differentiation in the presence of the notochordal process, which is not present in stage 6 embryos.

Decidua. The epithelial layer is intact. The glands are markedly tortuous (fig. 39) and lined by secretory epithelium. The stroma is edematous and shows a decidual reaction.

Chorion. The villi, which may reach a length of 0.5 or even 1 mm, are either present on the entire surface of the chorion (No. 7802, fig. 40) or are absent superficially (Biggart specimen). In one specimen (Hugo), 942 villi were counted (Stieve, 1926b). The mesoblastic cores of the villi contain vascular primordia which are said to be derived from (1) cells arising by delamination from the cytotrophoblast lining the chorionic cavity and then migrating into the villi, and (2) angioblasts differentiating from the cytotrophoblastic cells of the trophoblastic columns during the formation of early villi (Hertig, Rock, and Adams, 1956).

At this stage (in the Missen embryo) "the human placenta clearly presents a combination of labyrinthine and villous characters. It must be stressed that the main trabeculae, which we will call primary villous stems, were never free villi. From this stage forwards, however, it would be pedantic to avoid calling the lacunar system the intervillous space" (Hamilton and Boyd, 1960).

Secondary villi, that is, those "branching or arising secondarily from a villus or the chorionic membrane itself" (Hertig, 1968), are seen by stages 7 and 8. Their formation involves all the elements of previously formed chorion (trophoblast, stroma, and blood vessels). They lack maternal attachment, and their limited movement has been compared to that of seaweed waving in a sheltered tidal pool (*ibid.*). These free villi (in the Gar embryo) may branch as often as three or four times (Hamilton and Boyd, 1960). At the periphery of the primary villous stems, the cytotrophoblast has broken through the syncytial layer and, by lateral expansion and fusion, constitutes a thick trophoblastic shell (fig. 25).

Amnion (figs. 41–43). The amnion consists of two layers of squamous cells: internally the amniotic ectoderm, and externally an interrupted stratum of cells resembling mesothelium. Between the two layers, some mesenchyme may be

Fig. 33. Dorsal view and reconstruction of the left half of a stage 7 embryo, to show the general arrangement and the shading employed by Florian and Hill in their graphic reconstructions. Based on the Manchester embryo, No. 1285. The cloacal membrane is here included in the measurement of the length of the embryonic disc. The shading employed to indicate the epiblast (in the median view), prechordal plate, notochordal process (different in the two views), primitive node, primitive streak (in the median view), cloacal membrane, and the allantoic diverticulum and endoderm will be used again in subsequent drawings.

STAGE 7

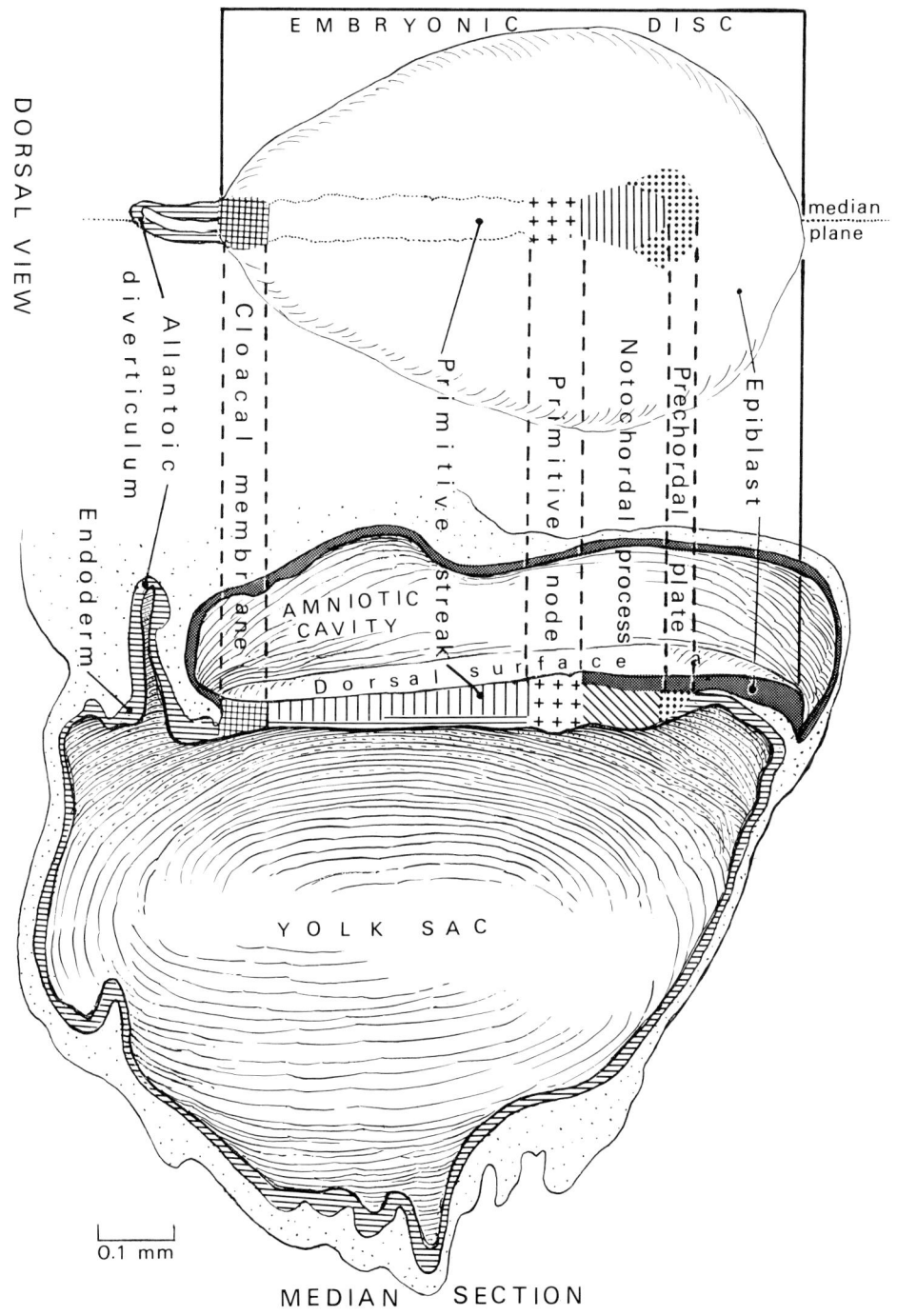

seen in places. An amniotic duct may be present (e.g., in No. 7802).

Embryonic disc. The dorsal surface of the disc is generally slightly convex (fig. 41). It varies in shape from oval (Biggart specimen) to piriform (Manchester 1285) but may be almost circular (Hugo, Schö).

Primitive node and streak (figs. 42 and 43). At the rostral end of the primitive streak, "the ectodermal cells are loosely arranged and . . . are disposed in a ventrolateral direction to form the primitive node" although a surface swelling is not necessarily present (Heuser, Rock, and Hertig, 1945). The primitive node (fig. 42), first described as a *Knoten* by Hensen in 1876, has been recorded as present in practically all stage 7 embryos, and varies in length from 0.02 to 0.1 mm. In some instances (e.g., Manchester 1285) the node appears to be separated from the streak by a slight constriction, or neck. From his studies of the pig embryo, Streeter (1927) regarded the node as an additional, specialized center and not merely as the rostral end of the primitive streak. The idea that the node appears before the streak has been discussed under stage 6. Intercellular vacuoles in the primitive node may presage the appearance of the notochordal canal (Jirásek, personal communication, 1970).

In the chick embryo, the primitive node has been shown to furnish at one and the same time the axially located mesoblast and endoblast (Nicolet, 1970). At the stage of the notochordal process, the streak "contains material destined for the formation of only the chorda, somites, lateral plates, and a small quantity of extra-embryonic mesoblast" (*ibid.*). Invagination remains active in the entire streak until at least the stage of the notochordal process, except in the node, where invagination has terminated already at the stage of the definitive streak (*ibid.*).

Although the primitive streak (including the node) attains its maximum length (about 0.7 mm) in stage 8, its greatest relative length (about 50 per cent of the total length of the embryonic disc) is probably reached during stage 7 (fig. 34). In the chick embryo, where the length of the streak is employed as a criterion of staging, the definitive streak extends over two-thirds to three-fourths of the area pellucida (Hamburger and Hamilton, 1951), whereas, in the human, it scarcely exceeds one-half of the length of the disc even at the height of its development.

The primitive streak is not necessarily straight, as has been shown in Hugo, Bi 24, and Manchester 1285 (Hill and Florian, 1963).

The presence of a primitive groove (which has already been seen in the previous stage) has been recorded in a number of stage 7 embryos, e.g., No. 7802, P.M., Robertson *et al.*, H. Schm. 10, and No. 1399 (Mateer). Its occurrence had been used by Streeter (1920) and by von Möllendorff (Meyer, 1924) in the grouping of human embryos. A primitive groove is never found in the absence of a primitive streak (Stieve, 1926b), although the converse does not hold.

Embryonic mesoblast. Mesoblastic cells accumulate ventral and caudal to the caudal end of the primitive streak, so that a temporary end node (*Endknoten* or *Sichelknoten*) may be formed, e.g., in Hugo (Stieve, 1926b) and in Bi 24 (Florian, 1933).

The embryonic mesoblast spreads laterally and rostrally from the primitive streak. Contributions to it are probably being made also by the gut endoderm and by the extra-embryonic mesoblast (Heuser, Rock, and Hertig, 1945). The limits between the primitive streak meso-

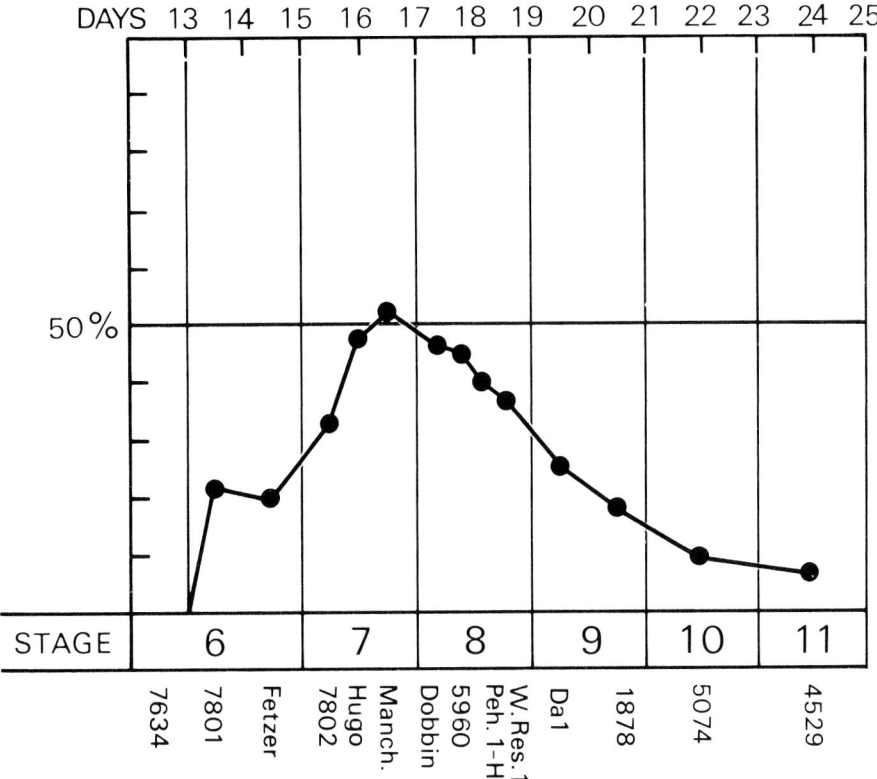

Fig. 34. Graph to show the percentage of the length of the embryonic disc occupied by the primitive streak and/or node during stages 6 to 11. Based on 14 specimens, which are listed below the graph. In the human, the primitive streak at its maximum development does not exceed about 50 per cent of the total length of the embryonic disc.

blast and the yolk sac endoderm are indistinct, and the two layers appear to be fused (Stieve, 1926b; Florian, 1933). In the Biggart specimen, according to Morton (1949), "in the angle between the anterior end of the shield and the yolk-sac there is a more loosely arranged mass of mesoderm which may well be the protocardiac area." As in the previous stage, localized mesoblastic proliferations directly from the disc epiblast have been recorded, e.g., in Bi I and in Hugo (Florian, 1945).

Notochordal process (fig. 41). The notochordal process has been said to be a prolongation of the primitive streak in the direction of the future head region of the embryo (van Oordt, 1921). The unsatisfactory term "head process" (*Kopffortsatz*), objected to by Waldeyer (1929a) who proposed *der kraniale Mesoblastfortsatz des Primitivknotens*, is better handled by the French authors, who write of the *prolongement céphalique* of the primitive streak. However, because the cell column "is without question primarily concerned with the formation of the notochord . . . it seems therefore appropriate to refer to it as the notochordal process . . ." (Heuser, 1932).

In the chick embryo, autoradiographic analysis has led to the conclusion that, at the definitive streak stage, all of the chordal cells are massed in the primitive node (Nicolet, 1970a), and that the presumptive notochord may be responsible for somite formation (Nicolet, 1970b). According to carbon marking experiments, the notochordal process does not form out of nodal epiblast, although it does arise in part from the rostral end of the nodal mesoblast and also receives contributions from the endoderm (Fraser, 1954). Removal of the primitive node resulted in complete absence of the notochord and in an apparent loss of control in the process of neurulation (*ibid.*). In the mouse, X-ray destruction of the primitive node area before the appearance of the notochordal process resulted in absence of the notochord, although a certain degree of cerebral neurulation occurred (Benoit, 1969).

The notochordal process, which is the characteristic feature of stage 7, varies in length from 0.03 to about 0.3 mm in the recorded specimens. In addition to a median cord, the notochordal process may also (in Bi 24 and Manchester 1285) possess lateral mesoblastic wings (Hill and Florian, 1931b). The notochordal process "very early becomes intercalated in, or fused with, the endoderm" (*ibid.*).

Although the notochordal process appears to develop from the rostral end of the primitive node, Hill and Florian (1963) had no hesitation in identifying the notochordal process in *Tarsius* before the appearance of a recognizably differentiated primitive node. This again raises the question, however, of whether the node may not actually be present before the streak.

The notochordal process comprises "not only the primordium of a part of the mesoderm (which does not seem to be very extensive), but also that of the chorda" (Hill and Florian, 1931b). The notochordal process, however, is not synonymous with the notochord, which does not appear until stage 10.

Prechordal plate. This localized thickening of the endoderm, situated rostral to the notochordal process, has been recorded in certain embryos of stage 7, such as Bi 24 and Manchester 1285. It has already been mentioned under stage 6 and will be discussed under stage 8.

Yolk sac. The cavity of the yolk sac tends to be slightly larger than that of the amnion. The yolk sac may project beyond the rostral limit of the germ disc (No. 1399), be approximately flush with it (Bi 24, Manchester 1285), or be receding in its relationship to it (No. 7802), although these variations may be due, at least in part, to distortion.

A yolk sac diverticulum may be present (e.g., in the Biggart specimen). In No. 7802, "detached vesicles observed in the chorionic cavity are regarded as transient parts of the earlier primary yolk sac" (Heuser, Rock, and Hertig, 1945).

The wall of the yolk sac (figs. 41–44), like that of the amnion, may be said to comprise, at least in many areas, three layers: mesothelium, mesoblast, and endoderm, from external to internal. Clumps of cells, especially in the ventral wall of the yolk sac, indicate that angioblastic tissue is differentiating. From their investigation of the Missen embryo, Gladstone and Hamilton (1941) conclude:

"The vascular spaces are partly developed by the fusion of small vacuoles, which are formed in solid angioblastic cords (intracellular spaces), and partly by direct transformation of mesodermal cells into flattened endothelium, which may either enclose the blood islands of the yolk sac, or form the walls of vascular spaces, which at first empty and incomplete, become secondarily filled with blood cells and enclosed by a continuous membrane."

Hematopoietic foci develop in the wall of the secondary yolk sac, although it is not clear whether they are derived from the endoderm or from the embryonic mesoblast (Hertig, 1968). It seems that they are definitely seen only after such foci are already present in the chorion and the body stalk (*ibid.*). Moreover, "it appears certain that blood vessel precedes blood cell formation" (Gilmour, 1941). From their study of the Missen embryo, Gladstone and Hamilton (1941) conclude as follows:

"The earliest generation of blood cells (haemocytoblasts and primitive erythroblasts) are formed in the wall of the yolk sac and in the umbilical segment of the connecting stalk in close connexion with the entoderm of the allanto-enteric diverticulum, and in the situation of the future umbilical vessels. A few rounded cells of endothelial origin were, however, found in the mesenchyme at the base, or amnio-embryonic segment, of the connecting stalk. These differ in type from the former cells which arise in close association with the entoderm of the yolk sac and its diverticulum."

Thus, although a number of workers have "suggested that the endoderm is the site of origin of the blood cells," nevertheless the blood cells may "depend for their normal development and haemoglobinisation upon their early release into the mesenchyme" (Hoyes, 1969).

At stage 7, three types of hemopoietic cells have been recognized in the blood islands of the yolk sac (Robertson, O'Neill, and Chappell, 1948): modified mesenchymal cells, hemocytoblasts, and primitive erythroblasts.

A low incidence of sex chromatin has been recorded in the yolk sac of No. 7802 (Park, 1957).

Cloacal membrane (figs. 36 and 44). The cloacal membrane is larger and better defined than in stage 6. It varies from 0.03 to 0.085 mm in length.

Allantoic diverticulum (figs. 36 and 44). Owing to the considerable difficulty in finding a convincing example of an allantoic diverticulum at stage 6, it is safer to assume for the present that the allantoic primordium first appears during stage 7, where it can be identified with a reasonable degree of certainty in such embryos as No. 7802, Bi 24, and Manchester 1285. In his discussion of the diverticulum of the yolk sac found in Peh. 1-Hochstetter (stage 8), Florian (1930a) referred to "the allanto-enteric diverticulum since its proximal part represents the later hind-gut, its distal portion the entodermal allantoic canal." In other words, "the very early primordium of the allantois does not arise directly from the hind-gut . . . but from an allanto-enteric diverticulum. The orifice of this diverticulum later comes to form a part of the hind-gut. It is only in the stage [10] when the insertion of the umbilical stalk has reached the ventral wall of the embryonic body that the allantois can be said to arise directly from the hind-gut . . ." (*ibid.*). This distinction was based largely on the relationship of the cloacal membrane to the orifice of the diverticulum. A comparison, however, of the wider choice of specimens now available would seem to indicate that, in stages 7 to 10, the diverticulum in question may be either allantoic or allanto-enteric at any given stage, as indicated in Table 13 and figure 35.

In the chick embryo, it has been maintained that the dorsal wall of the allantois is situated close to the epiblast, and the combination "appears to be the cloacal membrane" (Gruenwald, 1941). These

Fig. 35. The development of the allantoic diverticulum. In A (Bi 1 embryo, stage 6b), a yolk sac diverticulum is present, but it is not the allantoic diverticulum. In B (Bi 24 embryo, stage 7), an allanto-enteric diverticulum (A and E) has formed and the cloacal membrane (C. M.) is incorporated in its wall. In C (Manchester 1285 embryo, stage 7), an allantoic diverticulum is present caudal to the cloacal membrane. In D (Da 1 embryo, stage 9), after the hindgut (H. G.) has begun to form, an allanto-enteric diverticulum can be seen. The system of shading is in agreement with that shown in figure 33. To aid in making comparisons, the caudal limit of the cloacal membrane has been placed on the same vertical line in each of the four examples. It is probable that, in stages 7 to 10, the diverticulum may be either allantoic or allanto-enteric at any given stage, as indicated in Table 13.

STAGE 7

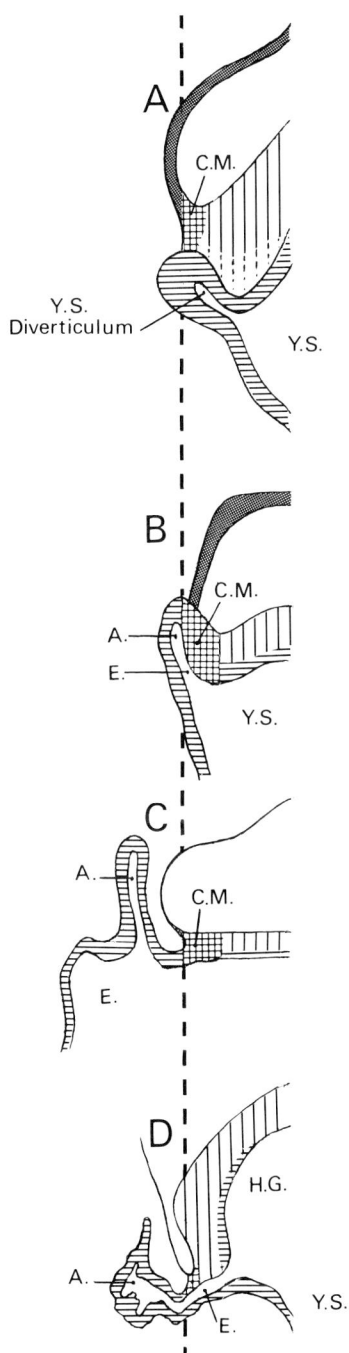

A+E = Allanto-enteric diverticulum
A = Allantoic diverticulum
E = Part of hindgut

Cloacal mem.
Endoderm
Primitive str.
Epiblast

(Median section)

TABLE 13. Examples of Embryos of Stages 7 to 10 Showing either an Allanto-Enteric or an Allantoic Diverticulum

Stage	Allanto-Enteric Diverticulum	Allantoic Diverticulum
7	Bi 24	No. 7802
		Manchester 1285
8	No. 5960	No. 8820
	Peh. 1–Hochstetter	Western Reserve 1
9	Da 1 (No. 5982)	No. 1878
10	Bi II	No. 5074
		Bi XI
		Litzenberg
		(No. 6740)

relationships do not appear to hold in No. 7802 or in Manchester 1285, although embryo Bi 24 (Florian, 1946, Plate 5, fig. 43) does seem to resemble somewhat the conditions found in the chick (Gruenwald, 1941, figs. 3 and 42) except that the hindgut has not been seen at such early stages in the human embryo. Embryo Bi I (stage 6) also bears some resemblance to the arrangement depicted in the chick but its yolk sac diverticulum is not regarded as the allantois. It would seem that Gruenwald's interpretation of the chick embryo is comparable to Florian's concept of an allanto-enteric rather than an allantoic diverticulum.

Primordial germ cells have been noted in the region of the allanto-enteric diverticulum in Bi 24 (Politzer, 1933).

"The essential part of the mammalian allantois from the physiological standpoint is its vascular mesoderm" (Mossman, 1937) and the question has been raised (George, 1942) as to whether "the precociously formed allantois in man may not have some inductor function in the origin and differentiation of the blood islands and blood channels of the body stalk." This would require the presence of the allantoic primordium by at latest stage 6b.

SPECIMENS OF STAGE 7 IN CARNEGIE COLLECTION

These are listed in order of serial number in Table 14. The list is based on the Carnegie records but the specific criteria for the stage have not been verified personally in the case of every specimen.

SPECIMENS OF STAGE 7 ALREADY DESCRIBED

(listed in order of length of notochordal process)

HEB-37. Summarized by Mazanec (1959). Chorionic cavity, 2.25 × 1.29 × 0.4 mm. Embryonic disc, 0.4 mm. Primitive streak, 0.104 mm, and node, 0.04 mm. Notochordal process, 0.032 mm. Yolk sac stalk (*ibid.*, fig. 77). Median projection published (*ibid.*, fig. 45).

H. R. 1. Described by Johnston (1940), who believed that a notochordal process (0.04 mm) and a prechordal plate (0.075 mm) were present. Florian in an appendix to the article disagreed, and his interpretation will be followed here (see stage 6).

Biggart. Described by Morton (1949). Curettage. Embryonic disc (narrow type), 0.27 × 0.16 mm. Primitive streak and node, 0.059 mm. A notochordal process is not referred to in the text but is mapped on a dorsal projection of the embryo (*ibid.*, fig. 2) and is approximately 0.04 mm in length. The specimen is said to resemble the Yale embryo.

Guá (Guálberto). Described by Lordy (1931). Hysterectomy. Chorionic cavity, 8 × 7.5 mm. Embryonic disc, 0.776 × 0.0465 mm. Primitive streak, 0.09 mm. Notochordal process, 0.045 mm. Possible notochordal canal. Said to resemble Hugo embryo. Probably belongs either to stage 7 or to stage 8.

STAGE 7

TABLE 14. List of Specimens of Stage 7 in Carnegie Collection

Serial No.	Grade	Fixative	Cutting Medium	Thinness (micrometers)	Stain	Date and Donor	Remarks and Reference
7802	Exc.	Alc. & Bouin	C-P	6	H.-E.	1940, A. T. Hertig, Boston, Mass.	Heuser et al., 1945
8206	Good	?	C-P	6	H.-E.	1943, A. T. Hertig, Boston, Mass.	
8361	Good	Bouin	C-P	10	?	1946, A. T. Hertig, Boston, Mass.	Abnormal
8602	Exc.	Alc.	C-P	8	H.-E.	1948, P. A. Younge, Brookline, Mass.	
8752	Exc.	?	C-P	10	H.-E.	1950, C. L. Davis, Baltimore, Md.	
8756	Exc.	Formal.	C-P	10	H.-E.	1950, D. R. Meranze, Philadelphia, Pa.	
9217	Exc.	?	P	10	H.-E.	1954, H. Jones, Baltimore, Md.	

Carnegie No. 7802 (figs. 36–44). An important specimen described and illustrated by Heuser, Rock, and Hertig (1945). Hysterectomy. Chorion, 3.75 × 2.35 × 2.2 mm. Chorionic cavity, 2.3 × 1.4 × 1.1 mm. Embryonic disc (broad type), 0.42 × 0.35 × 0.05 mm. Primitive streak, 0.11 mm, and node, 0.03 mm. Notochordal process, 0.048 mm. Presumed age, 16 days. Median projection published (*ibid.*, plate 6; Mazanec, 1959, fig. 46) and dorsal projection has been prepared by the present writer.

P.M. Described by Meyer (1924). Curettage. Measurements have been criticized by Stieve (1926) but defended by Mazanec (1959). Chorion, 3.9 × 3.77 × 2.5 mm. Chorionic cavity, 2.7 × 2.6 × 2.1 mm. Embryonic disc (circular), 0.41 × 0.41 mm. Primitive streak, 0.12 mm, and node, 0.02 mm. Notochordal process, 0.06 mm, acknowledged by Mazanec (1959) although denied by Fahrenholz (1927). No notochordal canal. Median projection published (Mazanec, 1959, fig. 47).

Hugo. Described by Stieve (1926b), who reproduced a photomicrograph of every second section. Hysterectomy. Surrounded by 942 chorionic villi ranging in length from 0.3 to 1 mm. Chorion, 6.4 × 5.9 × 5.6 mm. Chorionic cavity, 4.7 × 4.4 × 3.8 mm. Embryonic disc (broad type), 0.635 (Florian, 1931a) × 0.63 mm. Primitive streak, 0.245 mm, and node, 0.05 mm. Notochordal process, 0.07 (0.11?) mm (Florian, 1934). No notochordal canal. Prechordal plate probably not yet developed (Hill and Florian, 1931). Dorsal and median projections published (Florian, 1934, fig. 1; Hill and Florian, 1931, figs. 44 and 11; Mazanec, 1959, fig. 49).

A specimen (hysterectomy) described by Robertson, O'Neill, and Chappell (1948) possessed a chorion of 3.816 × 3.639 × 2.687 mm. Chorionic cavity, 2.718 × 2.239 × 1.679 mm. Embryonic disc (broad type), 0.462 × 0.485 mm. Primitive streak, 0.138 mm, and node (situated halfway), 0.03 mm. Notochordal process, 0.072 mm. Suggestion of notochordal canal in one or two sections. Assigned to horizon VIII by authors but probably belongs to stage 7. Median projection published (*ibid.*, fig. 12).

D'Arrigo (1961) described an embryonic disc of 0.47 mm, which showed a notochordal process of 0.075 mm. Canalization of the process is "doubtful" but the presence of a prechordal plate is "probable." The specimen "could be recorded in Streeter's horizon VII."

Goodwin. Described by Kindred (1933). Tubal. Chorion, 5.8 × 2.72 × 2.25 mm. Chorionic cavity, 2.44 × 2.25 × 0.75 mm. Embryonic disc, 0.588 mm in width. Primitive streak, 0.215 mm, and node, 0.078 mm. Notochordal process, 0.078 mm. No notochordal canal and no prechordal plate.

Pha I. Summarized by Mazanec (1959). Chorionic cavity, 7.872 × 5.475 × 2.032 mm. Embryonic disc, 0.66 × 0.52 mm. Primitive streak, 0.145 mm, and node, 0.06 mm. Notochordal process, 0.09 mm. No prechordal plate. Median projection published (*ibid.*, fig. 51).

H. Schm. 10 (H. Schmid). Described briefly by Grosser (1931c). Embryonic disc (almost circular), 0.51 × 0.58 mm. Primitive streak, 0.14 mm, and node, 0.1 mm. Notochordal process, 0.1 mm. Probably belongs to stage 7, although a cavity in one section was thought to represent "Lieberkühn's canal."

Bi 24 (Bittmann). Described by Hill and Florian (1931b). Chorionic cavity, 3.05 × 3.036 × 3.029 mm. Embryonic disc (narrow type), 0.62 × 0.39 mm. Primitive streak, 0.28 mm, and node (Mazanec, 1959, fig. 105), 0.05 mm.

Notochordal process, 0.105 mm, consists of median cord and lateral mesoblastic wings. Prechordal plate, 0.03 mm. Possible primordial germ cells in endoderm of region of cloacal membrane and in yolk sac endoderm caudally (Florian, 1931); Politzer (1933) counted 41 germ cells in the region of the allanto-enteric diverticulum in this embryo, and 19 such cells in another presomite specimen (Bi 25). Dorsal and median projections published (Hill and Florian, 1931, figs. 4 and 12; Florian, 1946, plate 5, fig. 43; Mazanec, 1959, fig. 50).

Manchester No. 1285 (fig. 33). Described by Florian and Hill (1935). Hysterectomy. Chorionic cavity, 4.28 × 3.28 mm. Embryonic disc (narrow type), 0.87 × 0.625 mm. Primitive streak, 0.39 mm, and node, 0.05 mm. Notochordal process, 0.125 mm. Prechordal plate, 0.03 mm. Connecting stalk attached to chorion at decidua capsularis (suggesting polar variety of velamentous insertion of umbilical cord). Dorsal and median projections published (Hill and Florian, 1931, figs. 5 and 13; Florian and Hill, 1935, figs. 1–3; Mazanec, 1959, fig. 52). Specimen is housed in Department of Anatomy, University of Manchester.

Pha II. Summarized by Mazanec (1959). Chorionic cavity, 4.985 × 3.882 × 3.52 mm. Embryonic disc, 0.895 × 0.62 mm. Primitive streak, 0.37 mm, and node, 0.06 mm. Notochordal process, 0.13 mm. No prechordal plate. Median projection published (*ibid.*, fig. 53).

A specimen described by Thompson and Brash (1923), which showed a notochordal process of 0.3 mm, is described in the present work under stage 8.

ADDITIONAL SPECIMENS

In the case of the following embryos, a precise measurement for the notochordal process has not been provided in the accounts of the specimens. They are listed in order of year of publication.

A specimen described in detail by Debeyre (1912) possessed a chorionic cavity of 5.6 × 2.1 mm. Embryonic disc, 0.9 × 0.6 × 0.95 mm. Primitive streak stated to be 0.54 mm in length. Chorionic villi (0.4–1.6 mm) showed some branching. Unsuitable plane of section makes it impossible to assess the specimen precisely.

Carnegie No. 1399, Mateer. Described by Streeter (1920). Hysterectomy. Angiogenesis in villi described by Hertig (1935). Chorion, 9 × 8 × 3.5 mm. Chorionic cavity, 6.1 × 5.6 × 2.5 mm. Embryonic disc, 1 × 0.75 mm. Primitive streak and groove present. Although the notochordal process was originally thought probably to be absent, Hill and Florian (1931) have no doubt that it is present. More advanced than Hugo (Florian and Völker, 1929). A very small twin embryo was originally described but that "interpretation has become open to doubt" (Corner, 1955). Drawing of every section reproduced by Turner (1920). A median drawing (Davis, 1927, fig. 5A) and a projection have been published (Mazanec, 1959, fig. 56).

Ho (Hodiesne). Described by Fahrenholz (1927). Abortion. Chorionic cavity, 6.5 × 6 × 3 mm. Embryonic disc (deformed), 0.6 mm (0.725 mm by flexible scale). Primitive streak, 0.22 mm (0.345 mm by flexible scale). Notochordal process just beginning ("undoubtedly present," Hill and Florian, 1931b). Possible prechordal plate claimed (disputed by Waldeyer, 1929a, but supported by Hill and Florian, 1963). "Lieberkühn's canal" (0.065 mm) is an artificial folding of the embryonic disc (Hill and Florian, 1931b). Dorsal and median projections published (Fahrenholz, 1927, figs. 32, 6 and 7; Mazanec, 1959, fig. 54).

Fig. 36. Dorsal view and median reconstruction of No. 7802, stage 7, in alignment. The dorsal view, which is based on a graphic reconstruction by the present writer, shows the location of the notochordal process, primitive node, primitive streak and groove, cloacal membrane, and allantoic diverticulum. The system of shading is that shown in figure 33. The median reconstruction is based on a drawing by Mr. Didusch (Heuser, Rock, and Hertig, 1945, Plate 6). A section of the allantoic diverticulum appears detached because that structure is not entirely in the median plane. The figure references are to the sections reproduced by Heuser, Rock, and Hertig (1945, Plates 4 and 5).

STAGE 7

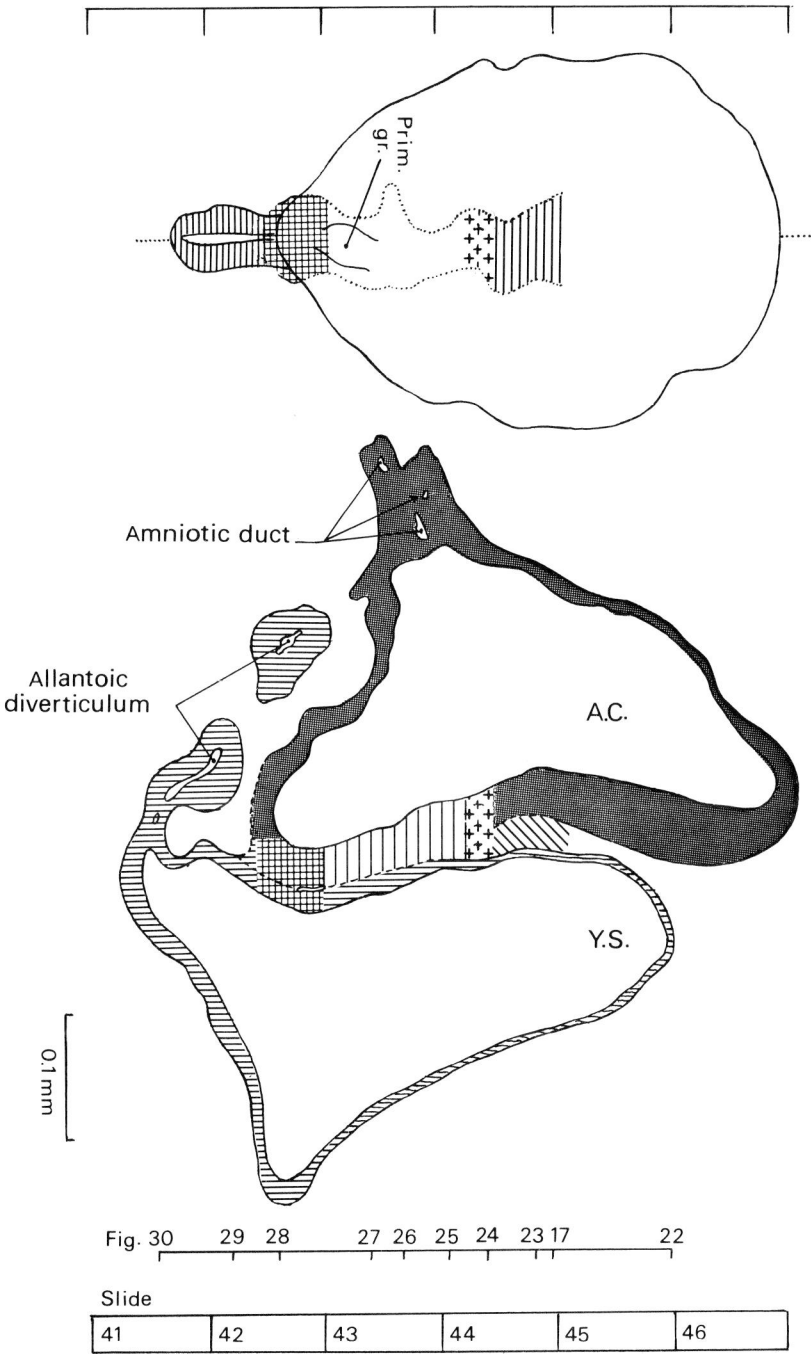

Fig. 37. Surface view of the implantation site of No. 7802, stage 7. Leakage of blood resulted in a clot which can be seen at the right-hand side of the photograph.

Fig. 38. Side view of the implantation site of No. 7802, stage 7.

Fig. 39. General view of the tissues at and near the implantation site (No. 7802, stage 7). A portion of the myometrium can be seen above. A cystic gland is present on the left-hand side of the mucosa. A large, branched vascular space partly surrounds the border zone of the specimen. Early decidua is present. Section 44-3-5.

Fig. 40. The chorionic vesicle of No. 7802, stage 7. The branched villi are evident. A cytotrophoblastic shell is forming. Section 44-3-5.

STAGE 7

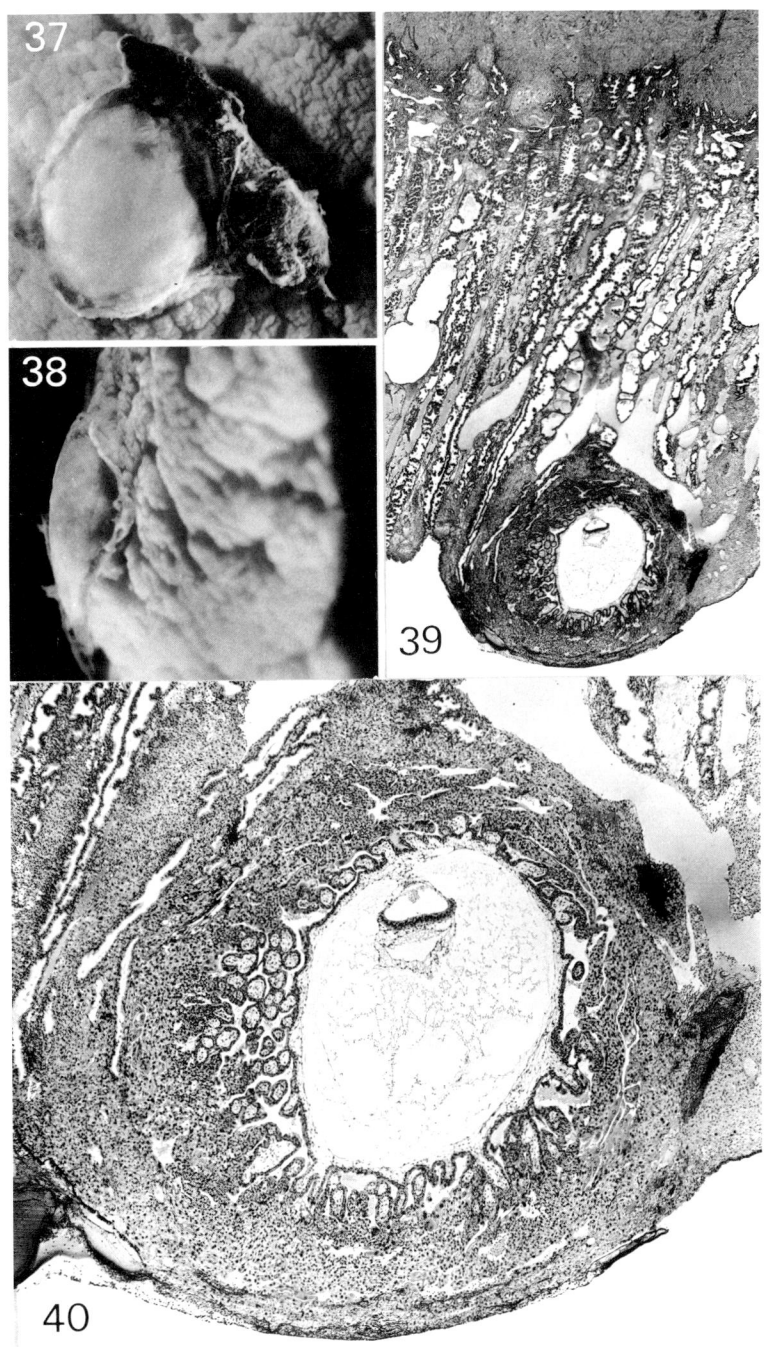

Fig. 41. Embryo No. 7802, stage 7, to show the notochordal process, which appears as a clump of cells underlying the middle of the epiblastic plate. Some intra- as well as extra-embryonic mesoblast can be identified. Section 44-3-3.

Fig. 42. Embryo No. 7802, stage 7, to show the primitive node, which appears as a rearrangement of cells in and ventral to the middle of the epiblastic plate. A surface elevation is not present here. Section 44-2-2.

Fig. 43. Embryo No. 7802, stage 7, to show the primitive streak, which appears as a group of cells emerging from the ventral surface of the epiblastic plate. The wall of the yolk sac is trilaminar. Section 44-1-2.

Fig. 44. The caudal end of embryo No. 7802, stage 7. A detached portion of the allantoic diverticulum can be seen above. Further ventrally, the caudal end of the amniotic cavity is evident, and the clump of cells in and on its ventral aspect represents the primordium of the cloacal membrane. The yolk sac is readily visible in the lower half of the photomicrograph. Section 42-2-5.

STAGE 7

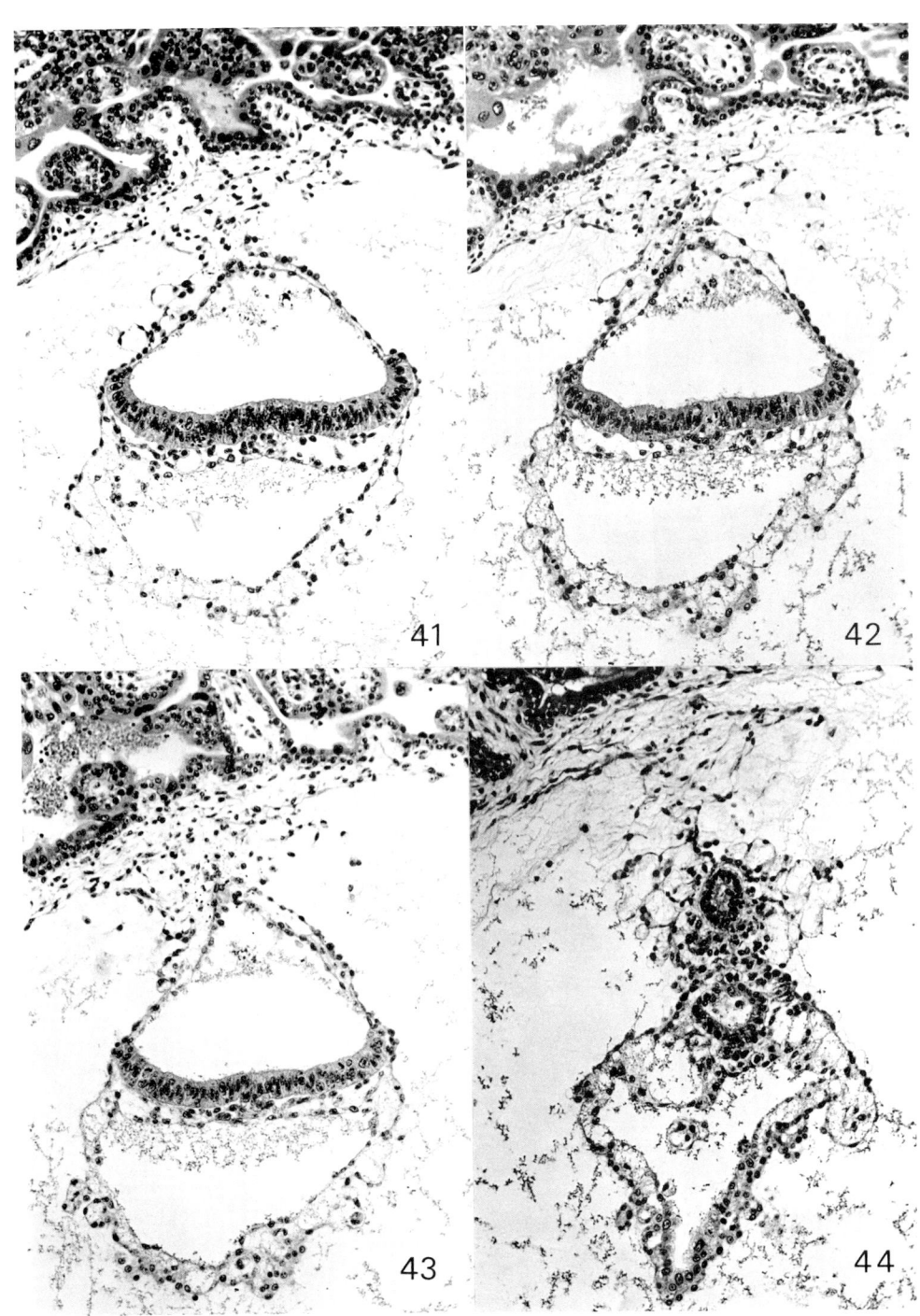

A specimen (0.9 mm) described by Debeyre (1933) possessed a primitive streak and probably belonged to stage 6 or stage 7. Large cells near the opening of the allantois were identified as primordial germ cells.

Falkiner. Described by Martin and Falkiner (1938). Curettage. Embryo damaged and not in good condition. Measurements seem too small (see Mazanec, 1959). Chorionic cavity, 1.5 × 1.4 mm. Embryonic disc, 0.15 × 0.29 mm. Primitive streak, 0.07 mm. Notochordal process contains "no definite lumen." Cells rostral to notochordal process are "probably" the prechordal plate. Development "agrees most closely" with that of Bi I. Median projection published (Martin and Falkiner, 1938, fig. 8; Mazanec, 1959, fig. 39).

Gar (Green-Armytage). Described by West (1952). Hysterectomy. Chorionic cavity, 3 × 2.6 × 2 mm. Embryonic disc (broad type), 0.56 × 0.69 mm. Primitive streak, node, and groove present. Short notochordal process. No notochordal plate. Said to resemble Hugo embryo. Trophoblast described by Hamilton and Boyd (1960).

Mal (Maliphant). Described by West (1952). Hysterectomy. Chorionic cavity, 3 × 1.8 mm. Embryonic disc (broad type), 0.45 × 0.6 mm. Primitive streak, node, and groove present. Notochordal process present (Mazanec, 1959); small cavity in node (West, 1952) or in notochordal process (Mazanec, 1952) "hardly sufficient to warrant the name chorda canal." No prechordal plate. Belongs either to stage 7 or to stage 8 (said to resemble Jones-Brewer I, which is a stage 8 embryo).

Carnegie No. 8602. Photomicrograph reproduced by Hertig, Rock, and Adams (1956, plate 10, fig. 53). Chorion, 2.73 × 2.43 mm. Chorionic cavity, 1.83 × 1.33 mm. Embryonic disc, 0.3 × 0.06 mm. Presumed age, 16–17 days.

Missen. Trophoblast described by Hamilton and Boyd (1960). Curettage. Chorion, 1.66 × 1.43 mm. Embryonic disc, 0.28 × 0.214 mm. Primitive streak and node. Notochordal process. Said to resemble No. 7801 and Edwards-Jones-Brewer (stage 6). Presumed age, about 14 days.

Certain other embryos that probably belong to stage 7 but that have not been described in detail will not be referred to here. These include Fitzgerald, Fitzgerald-Brewer II, and Jones-Brewer II (Brewer and Fitzgerald, 1937).

STAGE 8

Stage 8 is characterized by the appearance of one or more of the following features: the primitive pit, the notochordal canal, and the neurenteric canal. The embryo is presomite, i.e., somites are not yet visible. The maximum diameter of the chorion varies from 9 to 15 mm, that of the chorionic cavity from 3 to 10 mm (fig. 45). The embryonic disc is approximately 0.5 to 2 mm in length, and the age is believed to be about 18 days.

In Streeter's (1942) scheme, horizon VIII was characterized by "Hensen's node, primitive groove." Both these features, however, are present in embryos already assigned to horizon VII (e.g., No. 7802) and may even be found in at least some stage 6b specimens. It will be noticed, therefore, that the criteria em-

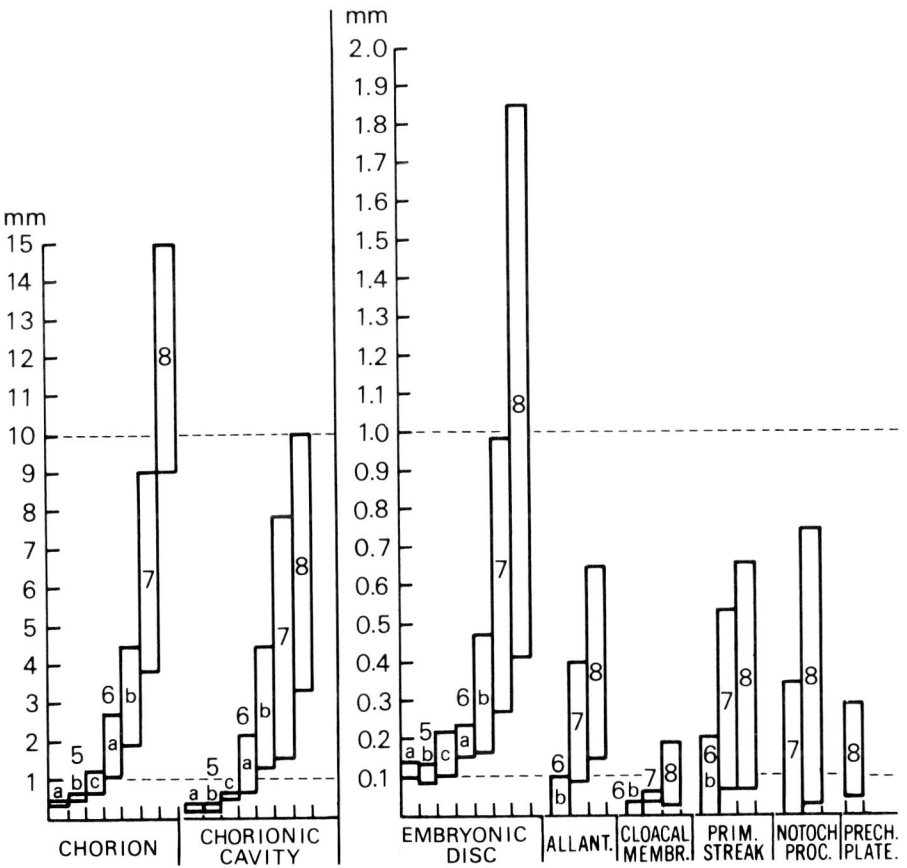

Fig. 45. The range of various measurements at stages 5 to 8. Based on 86 specimens (3 at stage 5a, 3 at 5b, 9 at 5c, 10 at 6a, 17 at 6b, 22 at 7, and 22 at stage 8). The two left-hand graphs are at a scale ten times greater than the others. It can be seen that the chorion attains a maximum diameter of 10 mm and the embryonic disc a length of 1 mm during stage 8.

ployed here for stages 7 and 8 are *not* those of horizons VII and VIII, respectively; a similar statement will apply to stage 9 and horizon IX.

By this time, the third week of development, the uteroplacental circulation is well established, the decidua well formed, and the decidua capsularis healed over the conceptus (Hertig, 1968). Very much later, namely, at midterm, the decidua capsularis will fuse with the decidua parietalis, thereby obliterating the uterine cavity.

A fairly high incidence of sex chromatin has been recorded (Park, 1957) in the notochordal process and yolk sac of two stage 8 embryos (Nos. 7666 and 7701, respectively), and a lesser incidence in the amnion, trophoblast, and chorionic mesoblast, whereas none was found in two other specimens (Nos. 7949 and 8727).

Although doubts may be raised in regard to certain other specimens, the following definitely belong to stage 8 and may be taken as representative of that stage: Shaw, Kl.13, Dobbin, No. 5960, No. 7640, Peh. 1-Hochstetter, R. S., Western Reserve 1, Gläveke, and Strahl. Drawings of No. 5960 are provided in figures 47 to 49.

Decidua. The conceptus is embedded in the stratum compactum, which is sharply defined from the stratum spongiosum (No. 8820, Jones and Brewer, 1941, plate 4, fig. 10).

The first maternal vessels in communication with the lacunae appear to be venules or capillaries, so that the circulation in the lacunae is initially sluggish. Moreover, "no direct arterial openings into the intervillous space are found in presomite embryos" (Hamilton and Boyd, 1960).

Amnion (figs. 52 and 56). The structure of the amnion resembles that seen in the previous stage. It is possible that "many of the cells of the amnion in the region of the peak undergo retrogressive changes and are sloughed into the amniotic cavity" (Jones and Brewer, 1941).

Embryonic disc (fig. 49). The dorsal surface of the disc is slightly convex.

With the exception of those specimens that are either broad (No. 8820, Schö) or particularly elongated (Dobbin, Western Reserve 1), the dorsal surface of the embryonic disc appears ovoid (Wa 17) or piriform (No. 5960). The interesting idea that two different types of young embryos occur was taken up and elaborated by Florian (1934a), who compared a "dwarf form" (*Zwergform*: Beneke, Bi 24, Wa 17, Western Reserve 1) with a "giant form" (*Riesenform*: Bi I, Hugo, Schö, Peh. 1-Hochstetter) at stages 6 to 8. To place this idea of dimorphism in mathematical perspective, the present writer has calculated an index (width $\times$ 100/length) for 65 specimens from stage 5c to stage 11. The result showed that 11 specimens had an index of more than 100 (broad specimens), one was at 100 (circular specimen), and 43 were below 100 (narrow specimens). Moreover, a gradual, relative elongation took place from stage 6 to stage 11. Specimens of stage 5c, which did not show definitive axial features, did not fit into the pattern. It may be concluded that Florian's study has served to emphasize that, from stages 6 to 8, wide variations in shape occur, and embryos may be squat or, more commonly, elongated. As in the case of bodily habitus in the adult, however, a range is found, and it would be an oversimplification to attempt to force all examples into Laurel and Hardy types. Both the embryo and the adult are pleomorphic rather than dimorphic.

The general area of the neural plate, comparable to that shown experimentally in the chick embryo (Rosenquist, 1966), can be visualized (O'Rahilly and Gardner, 1971). Indeed, areas for the probable location of the future epidermis, neural crest, alar plate, and basal plate may be envisioned in accordance with the scheme (Rosenquist, fig. 1) employed for the chick blastoderm. In amphibian embryos it has been shown that the formation of the neural plate is "induced" by the "chordamesoderm," Spemann's organizer (Jacobson, 1966; see also Landesman, 1967, and Toivonen and Saxén, 1968).

The neural groove (fig. 53) appears first in the more advanced specimens of stage 8: No. 5960, No. 7640, R.S. These three embryos possess a notochordal process longer than 0.4 mm. The neural groove (formerly called medullary groove) has been recorded also in M'Intyre and Gläveke (where the precise length of the notochordal process is not known).

The ectodermal cells, mostly tall and columnar, rest upon a basement membrane except in the line of the axial formation. The transition to the flat cells of the amniotic ectoderm is sharp. Cells in mitosis are frequent. Small, deeply stained protein coagulation granules are taken to be evidence of necrosis, which is said to be "noted in all normal young embryos" (Jones and Brewer, 1941). It may be mentioned in passing that cell deaths in normal human ontogeny have been studied chiefly in embryos from 3 mm in length onwards (Ilieş, 1967).

The endoderm is in close contact with the primitive node (Stieve, 1926, figs. 18 and 19). It presents gentle elevations and depressions as seen from the ventral aspect, and its dorsal surface, "due to numerous extensions which lead toward the mesoderm, has the appearance of a range of mountains" (Heuser, 1932).

In Bi 24, certain cells in the endoderm in the region of the cloacal membrane, as well as caudally in the yolk sac endoderm, were thought to be probably primordial germ cells (Florian, 1931; Politzer, 1933). Such cells, although sought, were not found in some other specimens, however.

Primitive node and streak. The primitive node has been recorded in most specimens. It varies from 0.03 to about 0.06 mm in length. The node may project above the surface, and it may (Nos. 5960 and 7640) be separated from the streak by a neck. In the intact embryo, the primitive node stands out as an opaque white spot (fig. 50). The node (fig. 46) may be merely indented by the primitive pit (Schö), possess some cavities (No. 8820), or be penetrated by a notochordal canal (Shaw). The cells of the node are large, possess more or less spherical nuclei, and tend to be arranged radially (Jones and Brewer, 1941). A plug (*Dotterpropf*) has been described immediately caudal to the dorsal opening of the notochordal canal (Rossenbeck, 1923).

The primitive streak (fig. 56) varies from 0.05 to 0.7 mm in length.

Embryonic mesoblast. Mesoblastic cells have by now spread beneath the entire surface of the ectoblast to reach the margin of the embryonic disc, where fusion with the extra-embryonic mesoblast occurs. The cellular density of the embryonic mesoblast is greatest near the primitive streak (Jones and Brewer, 1941, plate 5, fig. 11). Some mesoblastic cells are probably being contributed by the endoderm also (Heuser, 1932). Some isolated spaces are just forming in the mesoblast (in No. 5960) and, "from their position in the pericephalic region (figs. 6, 7, and 12) it is evident that they represent the pericardial cavities . . ." (*ibid.*). These spaces rapidly coalesce to form the

U-shaped pericardial coelom (M'Intyre, 1928, text-fig. 7). In an advanced embryo (Gläveke) of stage 8, the presence of "a true typical endothelial anlage" of the heart, situated between the endoderm and mesoblast, has been claimed (Evans in Keibel and Mall, 1912, fig. 404).

Notochordal process. The notochordal process, which varies from 0.01 to 0.7 mm in length, is fused with the endoderm and is in contact laterally with the mesoblast. As pointed out to the writer by Dr. J. Jirásek, cytodesmata may be seen between the notochordal process and the overlying disc epiblast. The fully formed notochordal process, as seen in the Dobbin embryo, has been described as consisting of three portions (Hill and Florian, 1931b): (a) the rostral part, an undifferentiated cell mass; (b) the middle part, comprising a median, canalized process and two lateral mesoblastic bands; and (c) the caudal part, which lacks the lateral wings but possesses the notochordal canal.

Notochordal and neurenteric canals. The notochordal (or chordal) canal (of Leiberkühn) is initially indicated (fig. 46) merely by the primitive pit (in Schö) or by some cavities in the primitive node (in No. 8820). In its typical form, it extends from the primitive pit into the notochordal process (in Shaw), where the cells of the process are arranged around it in a radial manner (fig. 57). The intact canal is of very brief duration, however, and the floor of the canal, which becomes intercalated in the endoderm, begins to disintegrate at once in several places.

It should be stressed that the term "notochordal canal" is used here for the canal in the notochordal process, that is, for the *Chordafortsatzkanal* or *Kopffortsatzkanal* (see Springer, 1972, for discussion), which is quite different from any cavity that may subsequently appear during the folding of the notochordal plate, an event that does not begin until during stage 10.

Already during stage 8 (fig. 46), in some areas (as many as seven in the Dobbin embryo) the floor of the notochordal canal may have disappeared (Kl.13, Peh. 1-Hochstetter, Western Reserve 1) so that the canal becomes replaced in part by a groove that opens ventrally into the yolk sac. Rostrally, the canal re-enters the tip of the notochordal process. The groove is situated in the notochordal plate, which is intercalated into the endoderm and, by increasing in thickness and breadth, appears to be more than "merely the remains of the dorsal wall of the chorda canal" (Odgers, 1941). Furthermore, "as Bryce and others have insisted, the breadth [of the plate] suggests that it must yield something more than simply the notochordal rudiment, i.e. that it probably helps to form the entoderm of the digestive" system (*ibid.*).

"It is probable that the disappearance of the ventral wall of the chorda-canal is subject to great individual variation, and cannot be used by itself as an infallible guide in estimating the stage of development" (Hill and Florian, 1931b).

The notochordal canal takes a course that goes from oblique to horizontal. With increasing breakdown of the canal floor, a vertical (perpendicular to the disc) passage appears (in Dobbin and R. S.) and is known as the neurenteric canal (Odgers, 1941). Both canals commence in common dorsally in the primitive pit, and the neurenteric canal may be regarded as the remains of the notochordal canal at the level of the primitive node (Van Beneden, 1899).

Prechordal plate (fig. 52). The prochordal plate is a localized area of endoderm which early becomes recognizable in that part of the embryonic primordium that is destined to form the rostral region of the head of the vertebrate embryo, and with which the primordium of the chorda early becomes continuous (Hill and Tribe, 1924). The term "prochordal plate" (van Oordt, 1921) has been used above as a synonym for the inadvisable term "protochordal plate" (of Hubrecht) but it is also commonly employed (Gilbert, 1957) for a more restricted area known as the prechordal plate *(Praechordalplatte* of Oppel). Another and unjustified term sometimes found is the "completion plate of the head process" *(Ergänzungsplatte des Urdarmstranges* of Bonnet). The prochordal plate, in its wider sense, probably does not contribute to the notochord but gives origin to (a) cephalic mesenchyme, (b) at least a part of the lining of the foregut (all or a portion of the endodermal layer of the oropharyngeal membrane), (c) the preoral gut (Seessel's pocket), and (d) the prechordal plate in a restricted sense (Hill and Tribe, 1924). The production of mesenchyme by the prochordal plate in the human reaches its maximum only after the differentiation of the somites (Hill and Florian, 1931b).

In *Tarsius* (Hill and Florian, 1963), at a certain stage of development, the thickened endoderm becomes arranged as an "annular zone," the rostral part of which is constituted by the "prochordal complex" (prochordal plate of earlier stages). In the rabbit, on the other hand, a horseshoe-shaped zone of thickened endoderm has been found, and whether or not it corresponds with the rostral part of Hubrecht's annular zone remains an open question (Aasar, 1931). In the human also, a horseshoe-shaped band of thickened endoderm has been detected by Hill and Florian (1931b) in some embryos of stages 6 (Beneke), 7 (Manchester 1285), and 8 (Thompson-Brash, Dobbin).

Either prechordal or prochordal, as used in a purely topographical sense, would seem to be suitable terms in the human embryo, and the former is employed in this study.

In most embryos of stage 8 the prechordal plate has been recorded as present, and it varies in rostrocaudal length from 0.03 to 0.3 mm. In No. 5960, for example, the plate (fig. 52) presents a very irregular dorsal surface "since cells are being given off to the surrounding tissue and some of them should no doubt be classified as mesodermal cells" (Heuser, 1932). Chromatophil granules (as described by Bonnet) and small, isolated cavities, or perhaps even a channel (Odgers, 1941; George, 1942), may be found in the plate. Although the prechordal plate meets the notochordal process caudally, it does not ordinarily reach the rostral margin of the embryonic disc. Further detailed studies of the plate in the human embryo, however, are needed (Gilbert, 1957). The difficulties encountered in distinguishing and delimiting the prechordal plate can be seen from the fact that, in the case of one embryo (Manchester 1285), Hill and Florian changed their view concerning its limits and, in the case of a second specimen (No. 5960), these experts disagreed with another (Heuser) concerning its location.

The possible relationship of the prechordal plate to certain types of tumors, such as epignathus, was mentioned by Adelmann (1922).

In summary, the delimitation and first appearance of the prechordal plate in the human embryo are not yet clear. It has been found in most embryos of stage 8, in some of stage 7 and even stage 6, and

Fig. 46. Simplified scheme of the probable modes of development of canalization in the primitive node and in the notochordal process. The notochordal canal is formed at stage 8 and extends from the primitive pit into the notochordal process (as in the Shaw embryo). The floor of the canal breaks down almost immediately (as in Kl. 13, Peh. 1-Hochstetter, and Western Reserve No. 1), and the neurenteric canal appears (as in Dobbin and R.S.). All the specimens shown here are human, with the exception of *Loris* No. 49. The neurenteric canal, which first appears during stage 8, may still be found in certain embryos of stages 9 (Da 1) and 10 (No. 3709), but not in others (No. 1878 and No. 5074).

STAGE 8

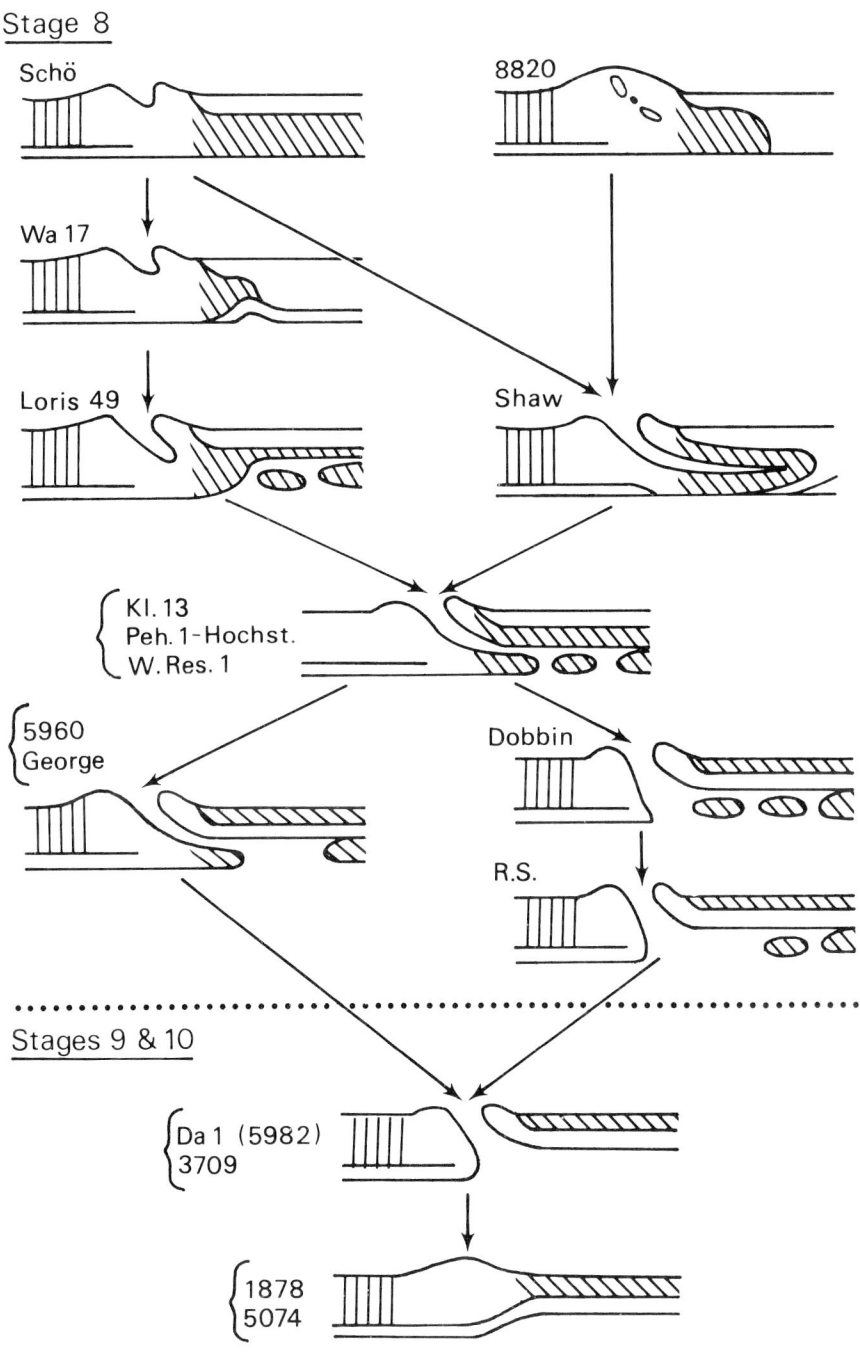

the possibility that it may be present at stage 5c has been raised.

Yolk sac. The cavity of the yolk sac is larger than that of the amnion. The yolk sac may project beyond the germ disc (No. 7640) or be approximately flush with it (Kl.13, No. 8820). The former relationship, however, is considered to be a distortion (George, 1942). Blood islands and blood vessels are seen in the wall of the yolk sac, and an occasional cyst may also be found. Mesenchymal cells, hemocytoblasts, and primitive erythroblasts have been observed in the wall of the yolk sac (No. 8820: Bloom and Bartelmez, 1940). A yolk sac diverticulum may be present (Kl.13).

A rostrally situated fold of the yolk sac (No. 5960) should not be mistaken for a precocious foregut. In more advanced specimens (M'Intyre, Gläveke), however, an indication of a foregut has been claimed to be present. An indication of a hindgut may perhaps be present in Peh. 1-Hochstetter (Florian, 1934b) but the assertion is not particularly convincing.

Cloacal membrane. The cloacal membrane varies from 0.02 to 0.185 mm in length. It has been suggested that "the cloacal membrane is early more extensive and that it later breaks down at the caudal end where the allantois is fused with the amniotic ectoderm" (Heuser, 1932). The primitive groove may extend onto the cloacal membrane, as in the Dobbin embryo (Hill and Florian, 1931b).

Allantoic diverticulum (fig. 48). Either an allanto-enteric (No. 5960, Peh. 1-Hochstetter) or an allantoic (No. 8820, Western Reserve 1) diverticulum may be present. It varies in length from 0.14 to 0.65 mm. Vacuoles may be found in the cells of the rostral portion of the allantoic canal, and have been recorded there especially in later stages (Hill and Florian, 1931b). The tip of the allantoic diverticulum may appear as a terminal vesicle and may even be separated from the remainder (*ibid.*).

Connecting stalk. The cells of the stalk are loosely arranged except in the proximity of the allantoic diverticulum. The stalk is covered by a layer of mesothelium which forms thin-walled elevations that may be mistaken for blood vessels (Bremer, 1914), as may also certain vesicles within the stalk (Hill and Florian, 1931b). Because the vascular network comes in contact with the surface mesothelium in some areas, the latter may be a source but not a very important source of vascular endothelium (Heuser, 1932). In other words, the mesothelium of the connecting stalk may possibly play some part in vessel formation (M'Intyre, 1928; but see also Hertig, 1935). Blood vessels are found in the wall of the yolk sac, in the connecting stalk, and in the chorion and villi. Two anastomosing vessels (in Dobbin), one on each side of the allantoic diverticulum, are regarded as the primordia of the umbilical arteries, and a possible representative of the later primordium of the umbilical vein may perhaps be present (Hill and Florian, 1931b). The future umbilical arteries are the first channels that can be identified as vessels having a recognizable course (M'Intyre, 1928).

SPECIMENS OF STAGE 8 IN CARNEGIE COLLECTION

These are listed in order of serial number in Table 15. The list is based on the Carnegie records but the specific criteria for the stage have not been verified personally in the case of every specimen.

STAGE 8   111

TABLE 15. List of Specimens of Stage 8 in Carnegie Collection

Serial No.	Grade	Fixative	Cutting Medium	Plane	Thinness (micrometers)	Stain	Date and Donor	Remarks and Reference
1399	Poor	Formal.	P	Trans.	10	H.-E. etc.	1916, H. N. Mateer, Wooster, Ohio	"Mateer embryo" described by Streeter, 1920
3412	Poor	Formal.	P	Trans.	5–15	Al. coch. E. au. or G	1921, H. G. Weiskotten, Syracuse, N.Y.	
5060	Good	Kaiserling	P	Trans.	5	Al. coch.-Eosin	1929, S. J. Goodman, Columbus, Ohio	Heuser, 1932
6630	Poor	Formal.	P	Oblique	6	H.-E.	1932, B. S. Kline, Cleveland, Ohio	
6815	Poor	Formal.	P	Oblique	10	Al. coch. or. G	1933, F. H. Swett, Durham, N.C.	
7170a and b	Poor	Alc.	C-P	Trans.	6	H.-E.	1935, A. T. Hertig, Boston, Mass.	Twins
7545	Exc.	Formal.	C-P	Trans.	6	H.-E.	1938, A. Plaut, New York, N.Y.	
7568	Poor	Formal.	C-P	Trans.	10	Al. coch.	1938, J. H. Meyer, Baltimore, Md.	
7640	Good	Formal. & Bouin	P	Trans.	10	H.-E.	1939, W. C. George, Chapel Hill, N.C.	George, 1942
7666	Exc.	Formal.-chrom. subl.	C-P	Trans.	6	H.-Erythr.	1939, G. W. Bartelmez, Chicago, Ill.	"H. 1515"
7701	Exc.	?	C-P	Trans.	8	H.-E.	1939, A. T. Hertig, Boston, Mass.	
7822	Good	Formal.	C-P	Trans.	10	H.-E.	1940, A. Plaut, New York, N.Y.	
7949	Good	Zenker	P	Sag.	10	H.-E. etc.	1941, A. T. Hertig, Boston, Mass.	
7972	Good	Alc. & Bouin	C-P	Sag.	6	H.-E.	1942, A. T. Hertig, Boston, Mass.	
8255	Exc.	Bouin	C-P	Sag.	8	H.-E. phlox.	1944, B. M. Patten, Ann Arbor, Mich.	Slides showing embryo returned to Dr. Patten in 1962

TABLE 15. List of Specimens of Stage 8 in Carnegie Collection (*Continued*)

Serial No.	Grade	Fixative	Cutting Medium	Plane	Thinness (micrometers)	Stain	Date and Donor	Remarks and Reference
8320	Good	Formal.	C-P	Sag.	8	H.-E. phlox.	1945, C. M. Goss	
8352	Good	Formal.	C-P	Trans.	8	H.-E. phlox.	1946, R. Choisser	
8371	Poor	Alc. & Bouin	C-P	Sag.	8	H.-E. phlox.	1946, A. T. Hertig	
8671	Exc.	Alc. & Bouin	C-P	Sag.	6	H.-E. phlox.	1949, A. T. Hertig	
8725	Exc.	Alc. & Bouin	C-P	Sag.	6	H.-E. phlox.	1949, A. T. Hertig	
8727	Exc.	Alc. & Bouin	C-P	Trans.	8	H.-E. phlox.	1949, A. T. Hertig	Germ disc folded, possibly double (Hertig, 1968, fig. 180)
8820	Good	Zenker-formal.	?	Trans.	10	H.-E.	1951, G. W. Bartelmez, Chicago, Ill.	"Jones-Brewer I" (H. 1459) described by Jones & Brewer, 1941
9009a and b	Good	Formal.	C-P	Sag.	6	H.-E.	1952, C. H. Heuser, Augusta, Ga.	Twins described briefly by Heuser, 1954
9123	Good	Formal.	C-P	Sag.	6	H.-E.	1953, C. H. Heuser, Augusta, Ga.	
9251	Good	?	C-P	Trans.	10–12	Azan H. phlox.	1954, M. Zeiler, Los Angeles, Calif.	
9286	Exc.	Formal.	C-P	Trans.	8	Azan	1955, S. M. Christhilf, Annapolis, Md.	
10157	Exc.	Formal.	P	Trans.	?	Cason	1967, D. A. Hansen, Salt Lake City, Utah	
10174	Exc.	Bouin	P	Trans.	8	Cason	1967, R. D. Martin, Odessa, Texas	

Specimens of Stage 8 Already Described

(listed in order of length of notochordal process)

Pha XVII. Chorionic cavity, 3.317 × 2.79 × 0.714 mm. Embryonic disc, 0.412 mm. This embryo is said to resemble No. 7802 (stage 7). In addition to a notochordal process (Mazanec, 1959, fig. 104) of 0.01 mm, however, it is thought to show probably the Anlage of the notochordal canal and an unusually large prechordal plate (*ibid.*). Possible primordial germ cells were seen in the wall of the yolk sac. Presumed age, 16–17 days. Median projection published (*ibid.*, fig. 44).

Carnegie No. 8820, Jones-Brewer I. Described by Jones and Brewer (1941). Hysterectomy. Chorionic cavity, 6 × 5 × 2.5 mm. Embryonic disc (broad type), 0.58 × 0.78 mm (in straight line); 0.6 × 0.79 mm (over curve). Primitive streak, 0.22 mm. Primitive node (0.06 mm) situated somewhat rostral to midpoint of embryonic disc. Three small, discontinuous cavities in node "represent the beginning of a neurenteric canal" which has no dorsal opening and does not communicate with yolk sac. Notochordal process, 0.0414 mm, but with no canalization. Hemocytoblasts and primitive erythroblasts identified in wall of yolk sac (Bloom and Bartelmez, 1940). Presumed age, 18½ days. Dorsal and median projections published (Jones and Brewer, 1941, figs. 11 and 12; Mazanec, 1959, fig. 48).

Shaw. Described by Gladstone and Hamilton (1941). Hysterectomy. Chorion, 11 × 4.04 mm. Chorionic cavity 8 × 3 mm. Embryonic disc (broad type), 1.05 × 1.34 mm. Notochordal process, 0.17 mm. Primitive pit and notochordal canal (which does not open into yolk sac) present. Prechordal plate identified but doubted by Mazanec (1959). No neural groove. Possible amniotic duct. Hemopoiesis (hemocytoblasts and primitive erythroblasts) under way in wall of yolk sac and in connecting stalk. Chorionic villi and endometrium described by Hamilton and Gladstone (1942); trophoblast further described by Hamilton and Boyd (1960). Presumed age, 18 days. Median projection published (Gladstone and Hamilton, 1941; Mazanec, 1959, fig. 58).

Wa 17 (Wagner). Described by Grosser (1931a,b). Hysterectomy. Chorionic cavity, 8.5 × 8.5 × 7.5 mm. Embryonic disc (narrow type), 0.98 × 0.7 mm. Primitive streak, 0.5 mm. Notochordal process, 0.18 mm. Possible dorsal and ventral openings of a notochordal canal. Prechordal plate, 0.075 mm. Presumed age, about 19 days. Dorsal and median projections published (Grosser, 1931a, figs. 4 and 3; Hill and Florian, 1931, fig. 7; Mazanec, 1959, fig. 59).

Kl. 13. Described by Grosser (1913). Traumatic abortion following salpingo-oophorectomy. Chorionic cavity, 8 × 6 mm. Embryonic disc, 0.67 × 0.5 mm. Primitive streak, 0.27 mm. Notochordal process, 0.2 mm. Notochordal canal, 0.25 mm (Florian, 1934) with dorsal pit and ventral opening: notochordal plate intercalated in endoderm. Possible prechordal plate. Presumed age, about 18 days. Median projection published (Grosser, 1913, plate 27, fig. 4; Mazanec, 1959, fig. 62).

HEB-42. Described by Mazanec and Musilovà (1959). Curettage. Embryonic disc, 1.17 × 0.72 mm; 1.43 mm by flexible scale. Primitive streak, 0.54 mm. Primitive node, 0.06 mm. Primitive pit. Notochordal process, 0.25 mm. Small cavity (primordium of notochordal canal) in notochordal process. Prechordal plate not mentioned. Presumed age, 17–18 days. Dorsal and median projections published (*ibid.*, figs. 1 and 2).

Dy (Dyhrenfurth). Described by Triepel (1916). Abortion. Embryonic disc, 1.6 × 1.04 mm. Primitive streak, 0.11 mm. Notochordal process and plate, 0.3 mm. Primitive pit, neurenteric canal, and neural groove believed to be present. Anlagen of hypophysis and optic vesicles claimed unconvincingly (plane of section unsuitable). Embryonic disc bent ventrally through a right angle (normality of specimen questioned). First somite probably not present.

A specimen (hysterectomy) described by Thompson and Brash (1923) showed a chorionic cavity of 10 × 7.5 × 4 mm. Embryonic disc (broad type), 0.68 × 0.9 mm. Primitive streak and groove present. Notochordal process, 0.3 mm, with no distinct lumen but notochordal canal about to appear. Mazanec (1959) considered that, on the basis of the reconstruction, the notochordal process could not be more than 0.23 mm. Definite prechordal plate (Hill and Florian, 1931b). Rough dorsal and median drawings included (Thompson and Brash, 1923, figs. 2 and 3) and median projection published (Mazanec, 1959, fig. 55). This embryo belongs either to stage 7 or to stage 8.

Schö (Schönholz). Described by Waldeyer (1929a,b). Hysterectomy. Embryonic disc, 0.99 × 1.03 × 0.11 mm. Primitive streak, 0.51 mm, and node. Primitive groove and pit ("indentation" is perhaps "first Anlage of [notochordal] canal"). Notochordal process, 0.34 mm. Prechordal plate. Said to lie between Hugo (stage 7) and Peh. 1-Hochstetter (stage 8) specimens. Dorsal and median projections published (*ibid.*, figs. 6 and 5; Hill and Florian, 1931b, figs. 6 and 14; Mazanec, 1959, fig. 57).

Dobbin. Important specimen described in detail by Hill and Florian (1931 a,b,c). Abortion. Chorion, 11.5 × 8.5 × 4.5 mm. Chorionic cavity, 9 × 5.5 × 2.5 mm. Embryonic disc (narrow type), 0.96 × 0.41 mm. Primitive streak, 0.42 mm to notopore. Notochordal process, 0.42 mm. Notochordal canal communicates with cavity of yolk sac by 7 openings, the caudalmost of which is the ventral opening of a very short neurenteric canal. Prechordal plate, 0.03 mm; rostral end of notochordal process was at first mistaken for prechordal plate. Dorsal and median projections published (Hill and Florian, 1931b, figs. 1 and 2; Mazanec, 1959, fig. 60). The scale in fig. 3 of Hill and Florian (1931) is incorrect (Florian, 1934). Specimen is now housed in Hubrecht Laboratory, Utrecht (No. H91; HH 159).

Carnegie No. 5960 (figs. 47–58). Important specimen described by Heuser (1932). Hysterectomy. Chorion, 15 × 14 × 9 mm. Embryonic disc (narrow type), 1.25 × 0.68 mm (in straight line); 1.53 × 0.75 mm (by flexible scale). Primitive streak, 0.5 (0.44?) mm. Primitive node, 0.2 (0.06?) mm, slightly caudal to midpoint of embryonic disc. Notochordal process, 0.42 mm (George, 1942). Notochordal canal (about 0.4 mm) opens ventrally. Prechordal plate, 0.15 mm. Florian (1934b), however, believed that the prechordal plate was situated farther rostrally than shown by Heuser. Angiogenesis in yolk sac, body stalk, and chorion. Angiogenesis in chorion described by Hertig (1935). Neural groove. Beginning pericardial cavities. Presumed age, 18 days. Dorsal and median projections published (Heuser, 1932, figs. 33 and 47; Mazanec, 1959, fig. 63).

Carnegie No. 7640. Described by George (1942). Tubal. Embryonic disc (broad type), 1.01 × 0.83 mm (in straight line); 1.16 mm by flexible scale.

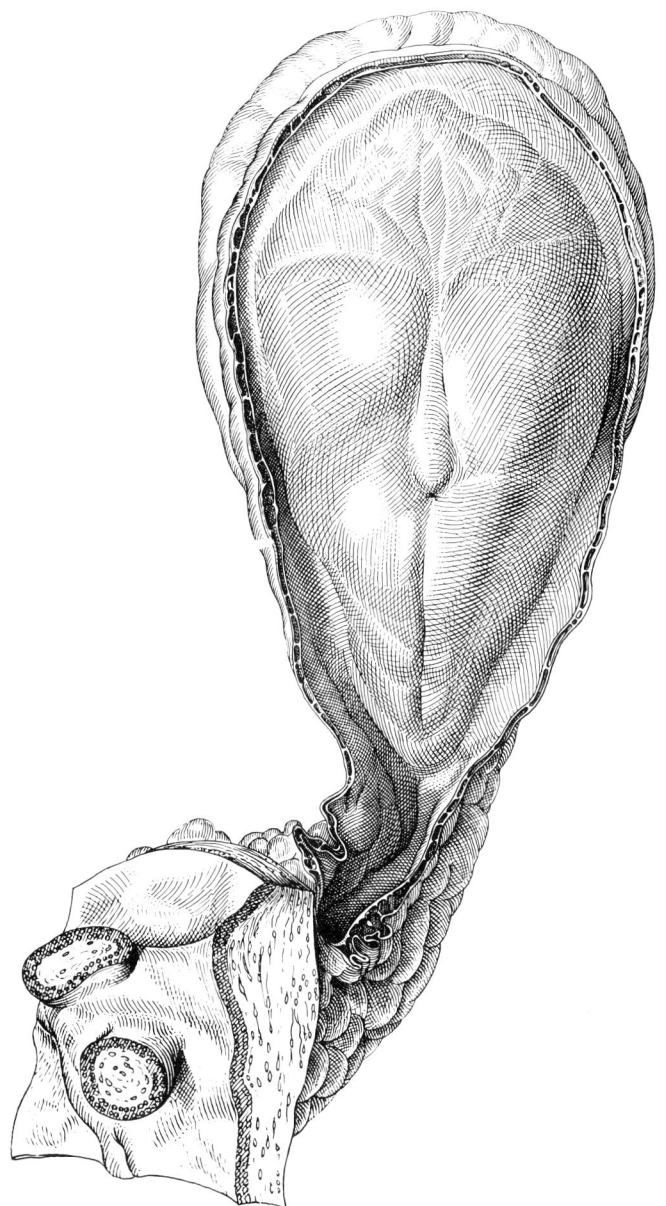

Fig. 47. Dorsal view of embryo No. 5960, stage 8, drawn by Mr. James F. Didusch from a reconstruction. The amnion has been cut, and, on the dorsal surface of the embryonic disc, the neural groove, primitive node, and primitive groove can be identified in rostrocaudal sequence. A portion of the yolk sac can be seen rostrally, and two chorionic villi appear in section in the lower left-hand corner.

Primitive streak, node, and pit present. Notochordal process, 0.44 mm. Notochordal canal continuous with primitive pit; floor of canal has disappeared in its middle quarter. Prechordal plate, 0.12 mm, said to contain continuation of noto-

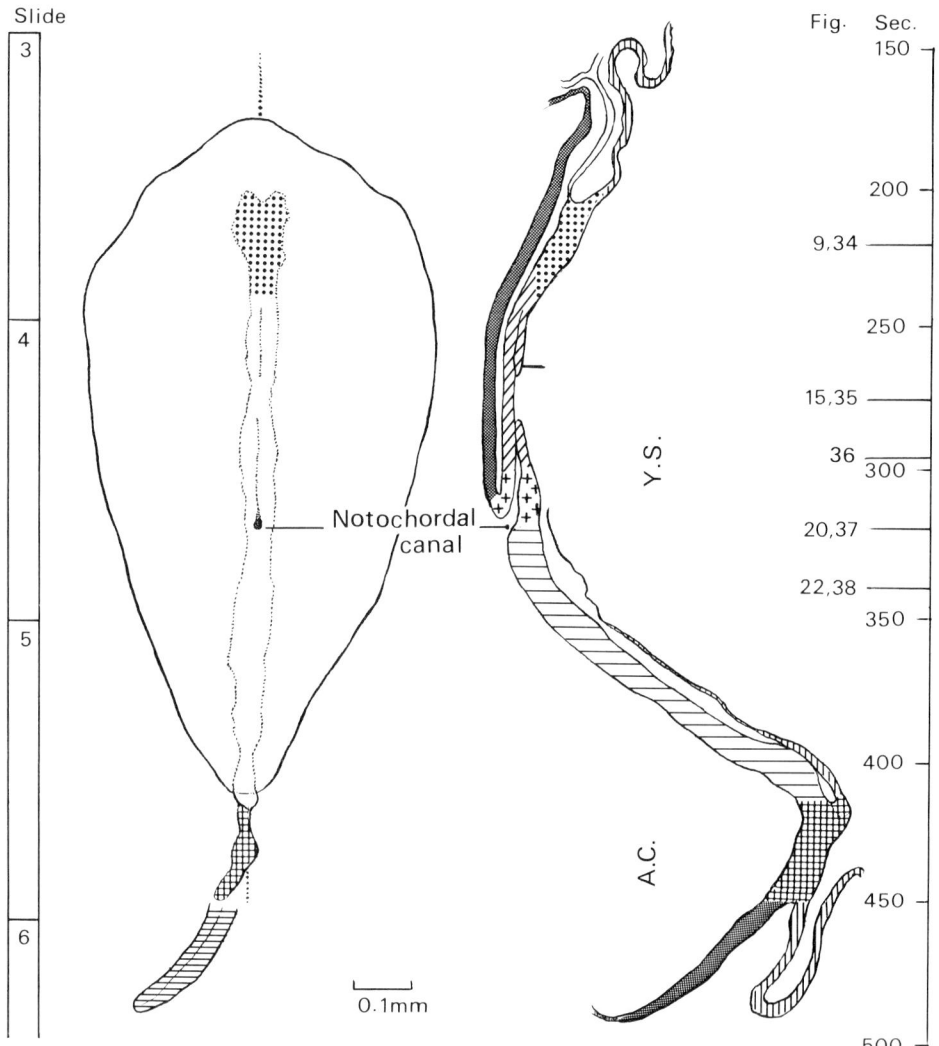

Fig. 48. Dorsal view and median reconstruction of No. 5960, stage 8, in alignment. The dorsal view, which is based on drawings by Mr. Didusch (Heuser, 1932, figs. 33 and 40), shows the prechordal plate, notochordal canal and primitive pit, cloacal membrane, and allanto-enteric diverticulum. The location of the prechordal plate is shown according to Heuser, and differs from the interpretation of Hill and Florian, who believed that the plate should be situated further rostrally. The system of shading is that shown in figure 33. The median reconstruction is based on a drawing by Mr. Didusch (Heuser, 1932, fig. 47). The notochordal canal can be seen to proceed from the primitive pit through the notochordal process, where the floor of the canal has disintegrated in its middle portion. Neither foregut nor hindgut is yet delineated. The allanto-enteric diverticulum can be seen caudally in close relation to the cloacal membrane. The figure references are to the sections reproduced by Heuser (1932, Plates 2 to 5).

STAGE 8

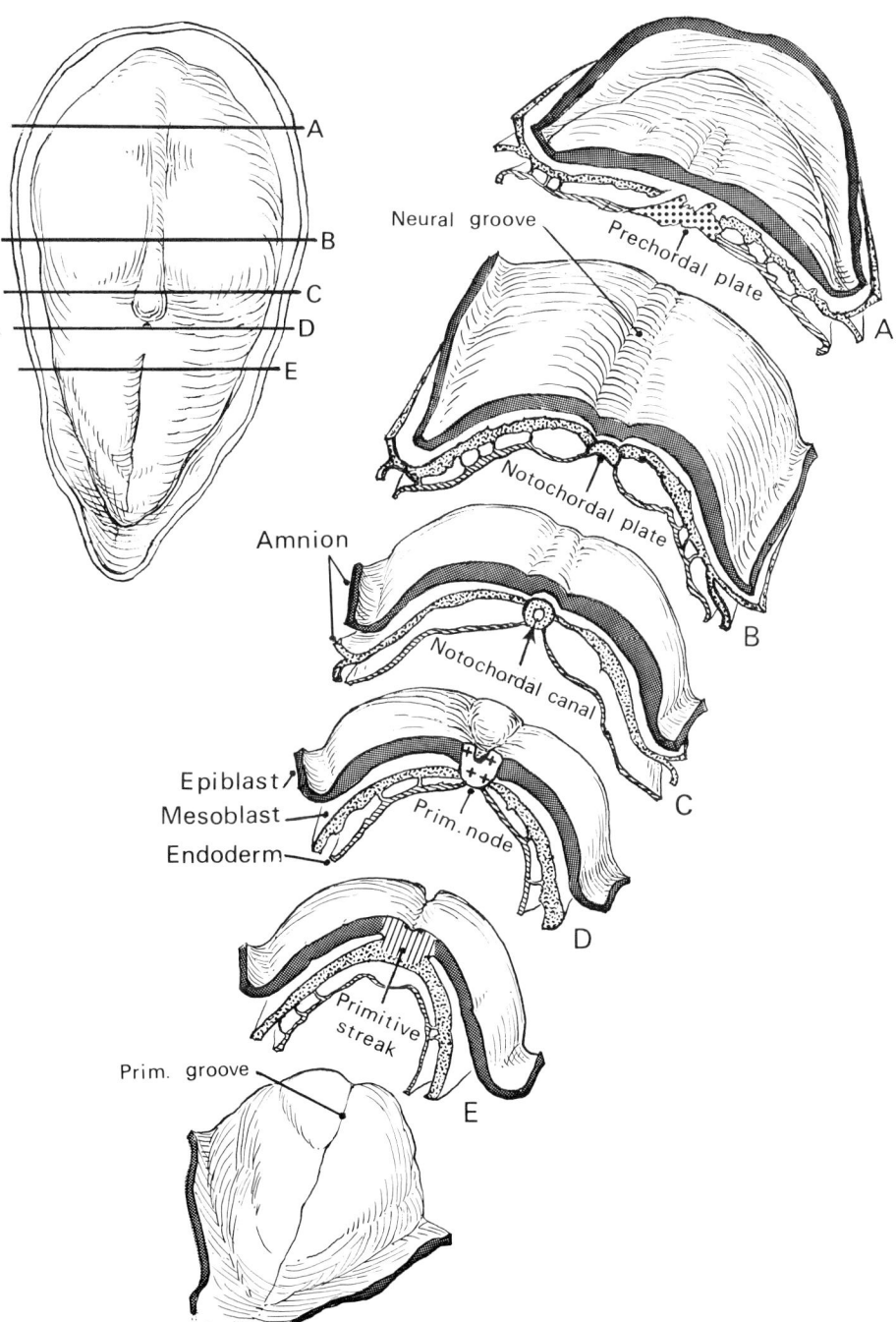

Fig. 49. Five transverse sections through No. 5960, stage 8, to show the arrangement of the germ layers and of the various axial features of the embryo. The levels of the sections A to E are shown also on a dorsal view of the intact embryo (inset drawing). The photomicrographs on which these sections are based are reproduced here in figures 52 to 56.

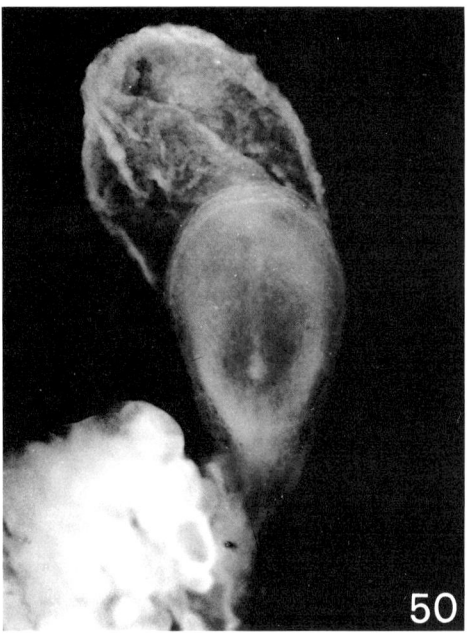

Fig. 50. Dorsal view of No. 5960, stage 8, photographed in formalin. The primitive node appears as a conspicuous opaque knot from which the notochordal process extends rostrally. The yolk sac is clearly visible in the upper third of the photograph, and the connecting stalk and adjacent chorion can be seen in the lower third.

Florian, 1931, figs. 9 and 16; Mazanec, 1959, fig. 61).

R. S. (Robb Smith). Described by Odgers (1941). Hysterectomy. Embryonic disc (broad type), 1.5 × 1.36 mm. Primitive streak, 0.4 mm. Notochordal plate (intercalated in endoderm), 0.7 mm. Neurenteric canal extends vertically from amniotic cavity to yolk sac. Prechordal plate, 0.29 mm, containing perhaps remains of notochordal canal. Commencing neural groove. Dorsal and median projections published (*ibid.*, figs. 1 and 2).

Western Reserve No. 1. Described by Ingalls (1918). Abortion. Chorion, 9.1 × 8.2 × 6.5 mm. Chorionic cavity, 8 × 7 × 5 mm. Embryonic disc (narrow type), 2 (1.87?) × 0.75 mm. Primitive streak, 0.67 mm. Primitive pit present. Notochordal process, 0.75 (0.65?, Hill and Florian, 1931) mm. Notochordal chordal canal. Neural groove. Dorsal and median projections published (*ibid.*, figs. 1 and 2).

Peh. 1-Hochstetter (Peham). Described by Rossenbeck (1923). Chorion, 10 × 7.7 mm. Chorionic cavity, 6.8 × 5.3 mm. Embryonic disc (broad type; this might be queried, however), 1.77 (Florian, 1934) × 1 mm. Primitive streak, 0.69 mm. Notochordal process (Mazanec, 1959, figs. 107 and 108), 0.6 mm. Notochordal canal ready to break through into yolk sac in one section. Prechordal plate (confirmed by Florian, 1931c), 0.08 mm. Indication of hindgut (Florian, 1934b). Allanto-enteric diverticulum (Florian, 1930). Dorsal and median projections published (Hill and

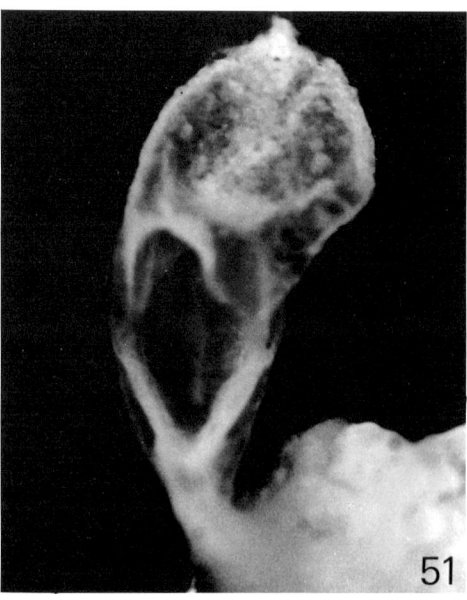

Fig. 51. Ventral view of No. 5960, stage 8, photographed in formalin. The notochordal plate can be detected. The yolk sac is clearly visible in the upper third of the photograph, and the connecting stalk and adjacent chorion can be seen in the lower third.

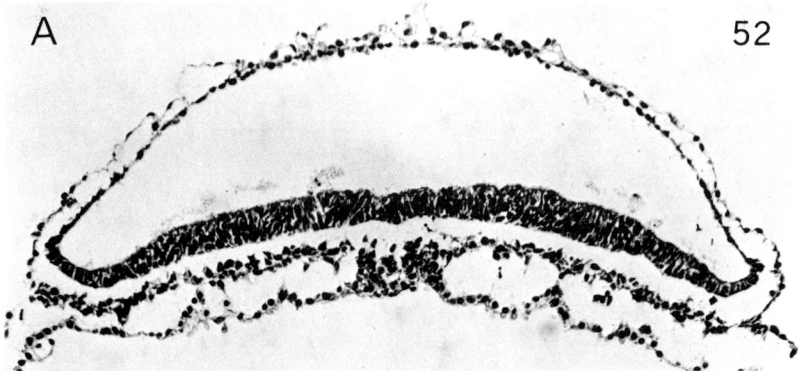

Fig. 52. The prechordal plate (Heuser's interpretation) of No. 5960, stage 8.

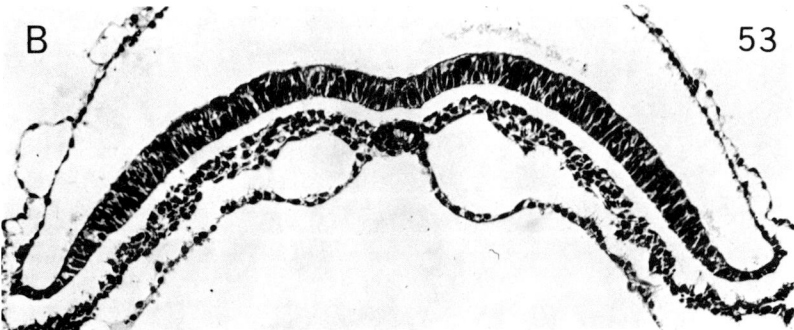

Fig. 53. The notochordal plate of No. 5960, stage 8. The developing neural groove can be seen.

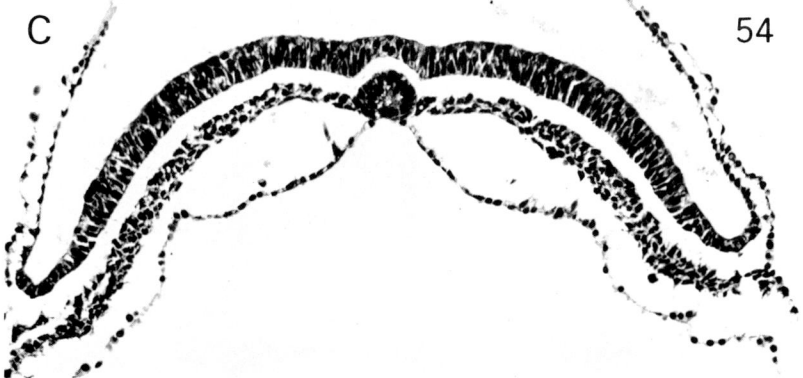

Fig. 54. The notochordal process and canal of No. 5960, stage 8.

canal, 0.34 mm, with three ventral openings into yolk sac. Prechordal plate identified (but not 0.4 mm in length, according to Mazanec, 1959). Dorsal and median projections published (Hill and Florian, 1931, figs. 10 and 17; Mazanec, 1959, fig. 64).

ADDITIONAL SPECIMENS

In the case of the following embryos, a precise measurement for the notochordal process has not been provided in the accounts of the specimens.

M'Intyre. Described by Bryce (1924) and M'Intyre (1926). Hysterectomy. Chorion, 14 × 13 × 8 mm. Embryonic disc, 1.37 × 0.5 mm. Primitive streak, 0.32 mm. Notochordal plate, neurenteric canal, and prechordal plate (with cavity) present. Neural groove, future foregut, U-shaped pericardial cavity, and "some general resemblance to somites" noted. Rough dorsal and median drawings included (Bryce, 1924, figs. 5 and 49).

Frassi's specimen (Keibel, 1907; Frassi, 1908) was illustrated as *Normentafel* No. 1 by Keibel and Elze (1908). Embryonic disc, 1.17 × 0.6 mm. Primitive streak and neurenteric canal identified. Neural groove. No somites.

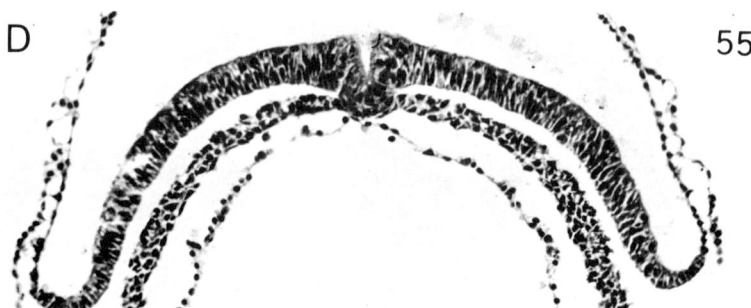

Fig. 55. The primitive pit and node of No. 5960, stage 8.

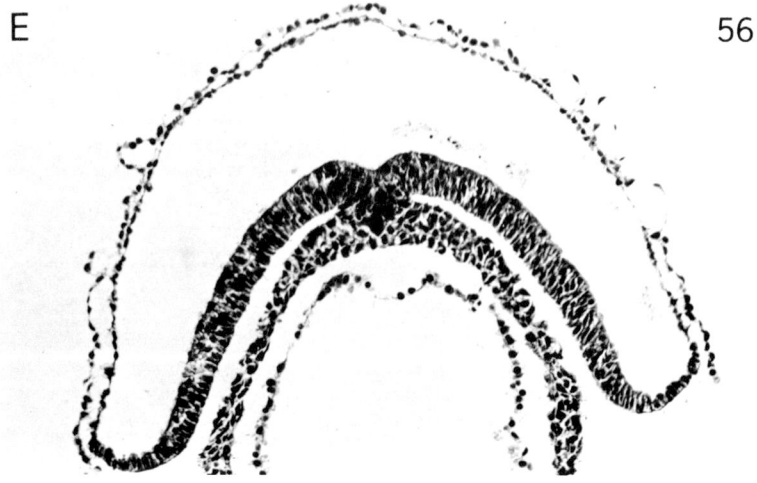

Fig. 56. The primitive streak and groove of No. 5960, stage 8.

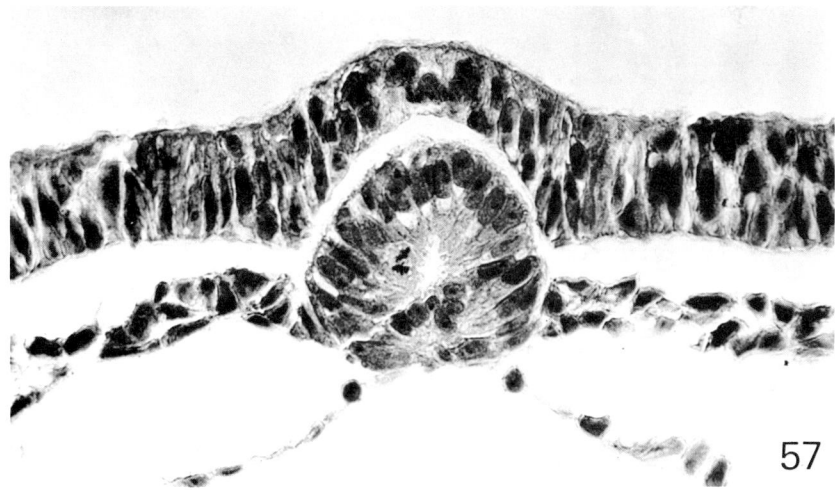

Fig. 57. Higher-power view of the notochordal process and canal of No. 5960, stage 8. Section 306.

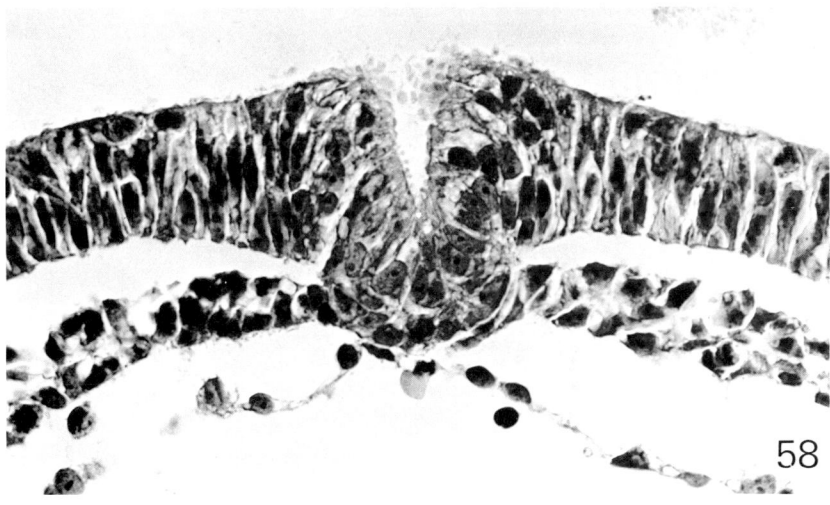

Fig. 58. Higher-power view of the primitive pit and node of No. 5960, stage 8. Section 320.

Gle., or *Gläveke* (v. Spee, 1889 and 1896). Illustrated as *Normentafel* No. 2 by Keibel and Elze (1908). See also Kollmann (1907) and Keibel and Mall (1910, 1912). Chorion, 6 × 4.5 mm. Chorionic cavity, 5.3 × 3.8 mm. Embryonic disc, 1.54 mm. Primitive streak and node, chordal plate, and neurenteric canal (Van Beneden, 1899) identified (see Keibel and Mall, 1912, fig. 231). Neural groove. Indication of foregut and pericardial cavities. Anlage of endocardium. No somites, although a small cavity on the left side (Keibel and Elze, 1908, fig. 4f) could be considered as the first Anlage of a myocoele.

A specimen described briefly by Strahl (1916) possessed a notochordal process and canal, and apparently a prechordal plate. A median drawing was included (*ibid.*, fig. a) but measurements were not provided.

Vuill., or *Vulliet*. Illustrated schematically by Eternod (1899a and 1909), Kollmann (1907), and Keibel and Mall (1912). Chorion, 10 × 8.2 × 6 mm. Chorionic cavity, 9 × 7.2 × 5 mm. Embryonic disc, 1.3 mm. Notochordal and neurenteric canals (Eternod, 1899b).

Carnegie No. 9009. Described briefly in an abstract by Heuser (1954). Hysterectomy. Monozygotic twin embryos. Embryonic discs, 0.9 and 0.66 mm. In each: primitive node in middle of disc, notochordal process with first evidence of canal formation. Assigned to horizon VIII by Heuser, who estimated the age as 17 days.

Carnegie No. 8671. Low power photomicrographs reproduced by Hertig (1968, figs. 47 and 181).

Carnegie No. 8727. Photomicrograph reproduced by Hertig (1968, fig. 180). The partial duplication of the germ disc shown in this specimen would presumably have resulted in conjoined twins.

Certain other embryos that probably belong to stage 8 but that have not been described in adequate detail will not be referred to here. These include Krukenberg (1922) and Fitzgerald-Brewer I (Brewer and Fitzgerald, 1937). Boerner-Patzelt and Schwarzacher (1923) described an unsatisfactory specimen (embryonic disc, 0.47 × 0.43 mm) that showed a neurenteric canal. Broman (1936) described in detail an abnormal specimen ("Lqt") in which the primitive streak showed "overgrowth" in relation to the neurenteric canal, resulting in a dislocation within the embryonic disc.

STAGE 9

Embryos of stage 9 vary from approximately 1.5 to 3 mm in length, and are believed to be about 20 days in age. Now that the neural groove and the first somites are present, the "embryo proper" may be said to have been formed (Van Oordt, 1921). At this point, it may be convenient to summarize graphically the criteria employed in distinguishing stages 5 to 9 (fig. 59).

The characteristic feature of stage 9 is the appearance of from 1 to 3 pairs of somites. At a certain period in vertebrate development, the number of pairs of somites that are clearly visible constitutes a simple and fairly accurate criterion for staging. Thus, in *Ambystoma maculatum*, stages 17 to 23 of Harrison show 1 to 6 somite pairs, respectively (Wilens, 1969). In *Gallus domesticus*, a stage has been assigned to every third pair of somites that is added: stage 7, 1 pair; stage 8, 4 pairs; stage 9, 7 pairs; etc. (Hamburger and Hamilton, 1951). In the human, greater spans of somite pairs have been assigned to each stage. Thus, after the first 3 pairs have appeared at stage 9, stage 10 shows 4 to 12 pairs (Heuser and Corner, 1957), stage 11 presents 13 to 20 pairs, and stage 12 possesses 21 to 29 pairs (Streeter, 1942), after which time counting becomes more difficult and other criteria are emphasized.

Although the degree of development is in general agreement with the number of somites, exceptions do occur. Thus, Davis (1927) found that the heart of a certain 4-somite (hence stage 10) embryo (No. 3709) was less advanced than that of No. 1878, which possesses 2–3 somite pairs and belongs to stage 9. It is of interest to note also that, in the central nervous system of chick embryos, it was found impracticable to relate growth to somite development, which latter showed a greater consistency with respect to time (di Virgilio, Lavenda, and Worden, 1967). Similarly, in the rabbit embryo, it was concluded that "the best criterion is a general survey of the degree of development of the structures present" (Aasar, 1931).

In Streeter's (1942) scheme, horizon IX was characterized by "neural folds, elongated notochord." The neural folds, however, appear during stage 8 (O'Rahilly and Gardner, 1971). Moreover, now that horizon X ("early somites present," Streeter, 1942) has been limited specifically to "4 to 12 somites" (Heuser and Corner, 1957), it follows that the first three pairs of somites must appear earlier, namely, during stage 9.

Stages 1 to 3 are sometimes referred to as pre-implantation stages, stage 5 as previllous, stages 6 to 8 as presomite, and stage 9 to approximately stage 13 as somite stages.

Embryos of stage 9 are very rare. Fortunately two have been described in considerable detail (figs. 60 and 63). A great need exists, however, for further thorough accounts of specimens of excellent quality.

Amnion. An amniotic duct may be present (No. 1878).

External form. As seen from the dorsal aspect, the embryo is frequently described as shaped like the sole of a shoe (fig. 61).

Many, perhaps most, embryos of stages 9 and 10 display a dorsal concavity ("lordosis") which has been subject to considerable discussion (fig. 62). Although abrupt bends and kinks are arti-

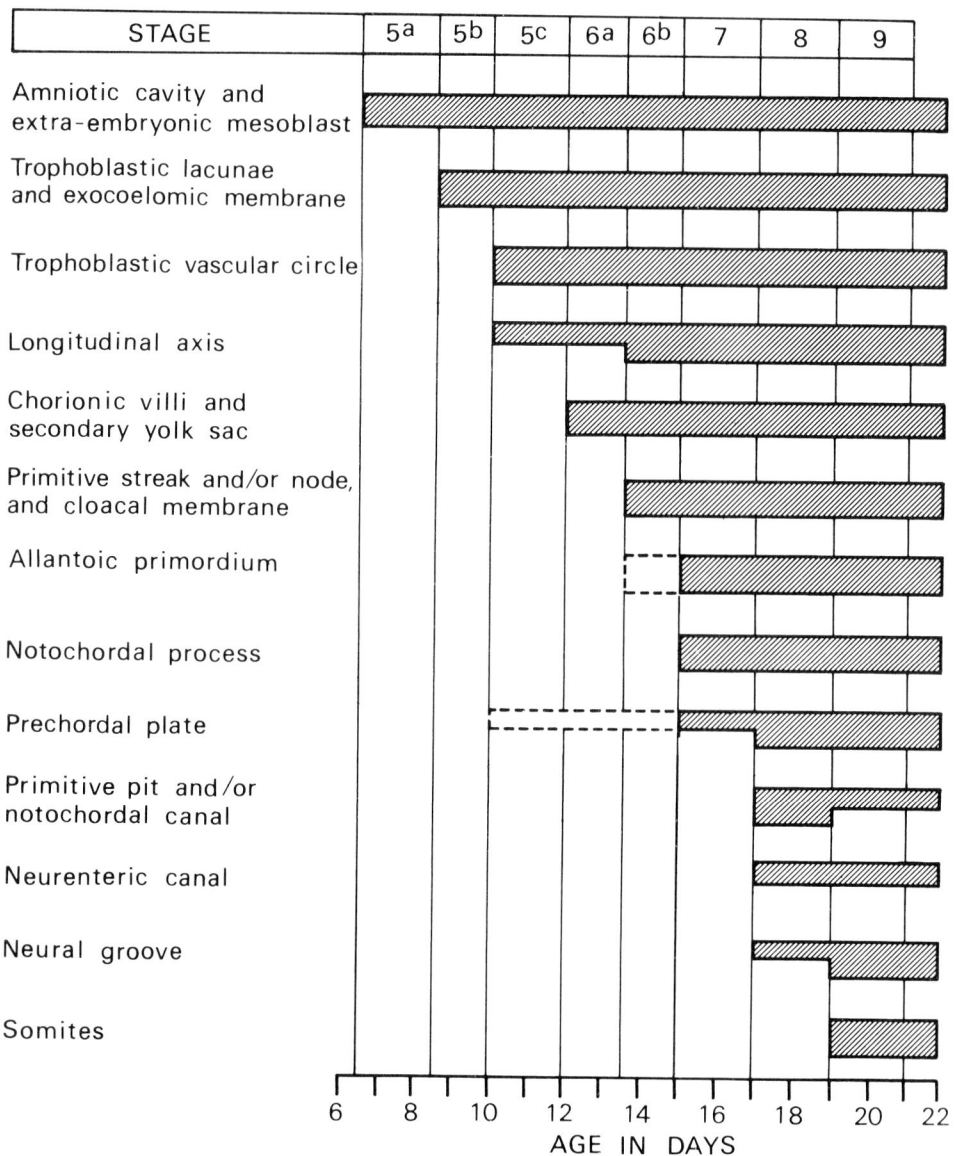

Fig. 59. Summary of the criteria employed in distinguishing stages 5 to 9. The shaded bars indicate the stages at which a given feature is found. The following are not used: appearance of amniotic cavity, appearance of yolk sac, branching of chorionic villi, cloacal membrane, allantoic diverticulum, prechordal plate, neural groove and neural folds.

facts, "anything from a gentle convexity to a moderate dorsal concavity must be considered normal" (Heuser and Corner, 1957). An excellent example can be seen in figure 66. At stage 9, the rostral and caudal ends of the embryo begin to be elevated "above" (dorsal to) the level of the yolk sac. It should be kept in mind, however, that a dorsal concavity is augmented by the collapse of the yolk sac; indeed, wrinkling of the yolk sac and dorsal flexure increase *pari passu* during dehydration (Bartelmez and Evans, 1926).

Although an indication of a head fold may perhaps be detectable in a few embryos of stage 8, the caudal fold does not appear until during stage 9 (in embryo Da 1). With the continuing elevation of the neural folds, lateral limiting sulci appear at first rostrally and then in the caudal part of the embryo (Da 1).

Studies of the chick embryo have led to the conclusion that "detachment of the head from the blastoderm is brought about to a lesser degree by independent head-fold formation, and to a greater degree by an influence of the fast growing brain. Presence of detached fore-gut is a necessary prerequisite for head detachment" (Gruenwald, 1941). Moreover, "we must abandon the conception of a simple folding of the blastoderm as the cause of detachment" not only for the rostral but also for the caudal end of the body and the corresponding gut. "However, the process at the posterior [caudal] end is entirely different from that found in the head region. Here, too, the detachment is most probably due to growth of the body beyond its attachment to the blastoderm" (*ibid.*).

Nervous system. Stage 9 heralds the onset of that developmental phase (largely stage 10) during which the neural folds dominate the external picture. The neural groove, which appeared during stage 8, is now quite deep although it is still open throughout its entire extent (fig. 61). About one-half of the longitudinal extent of the groove represents the future brain. The area of the forebrain is conspicuous, and its neural folds are separated rostrally from each other by the terminal notch, which leads to the oropharyngeal membrane. Although comparison with the more advanced embryos of stage 10 allows the approximate site of the future optic sulci to be determined, optic primordia are not yet visible.

In the more advanced specimens of stage 9, the neural axis, at the caudal end of the forebrain, changes its direction through an angle of about 115 degrees (in No. 1878). This alteration of axis constitutes the cranial (or mesencephalic) flexure, which, in this and subsequent stages, occurs at the midbrain (fig. 62). The flexure is probably the result of the more rapid growth of the dorsal, as compared with the ventral, lamina of the midbrain (Bartelmez and Evans, 1926).

A distinct isthmus separates the midbrain from the hindbrain. The latter comprises three rhombomeres.[1]

The interval between the summits of the neural folds is narrowest in the junctional region between hindbrain and future spinal cord, and it is here that closure of the neural groove will first take place during stage 10.

The otic disc (or plate) makes its appearance during stage 9 (fig. 64). At first ill defined and merely suggested (Ludwig, 1928, fig. 9), it is soon (O'Rahilly, 1963) a better marked ectodermal thickening (in No. 1878; fig. 64) approximately opposite the middle of the rhombencephalic fold. The otic disc probably involves more ectoderm than is eventually incorporated into the otic vesicle (Bartelmez and Evans, 1926). A cellular collection nearby has been claimed to be perhaps the primordium of the trigeminal ganglion (Ingalls, 1920), although neural

---

[1] In the terminology of Bergquist and Källén (personal communication, 1969), the hindbrain comprises three "proneuromeres" (C, D, and E), each of which may subsequently be divided into neuromeres (d and e; f and g; h and i). For other viewpoints on neuromery, see Vaage (1969).

crest in general has not been identified in the human embryo until stage 10.

The head ectoderm is undergoing differentiation such that several areas (fig. 62) have been mapped out in one specimen (Bartelmez and Evans, 1926, plate 3, fig. 3): the otic disc (already mentioned); the trigeminal nerve area; the ectodermal area that will later cover the hyoid (second pharyngeal) arch; and the site of the first pharyngeal membrane (overlying the first pharyngeal pouch).

Gut. The foregut develops during stage 9 (or possibly at the end of stage 8) as a recess of the yolk sac. The midgut and hindgut, however, are either still combined (No. 1878 and No. 5080) or else (fig. 60) the hindgut is making its appearance as a separate recess (Da 1). In the former case, the cloacal membrane is as yet in the roof of the gut and, just caudal to it, the allantoic diverticulum arises (fig. 63). In brief, although a rostral intestinal portal is present at this stage, a caudal portal may or may not be. In an excellent specimen not yet published (Prague No. 2008; 3 somite pairs; embryonic disc, 1.73 mm), which the present writer examined through the kindness of Dr. J. E. Jirásek, the caudal fold, the hindgut, the caudal intestinal portal, and caudal coelomic cavities are all well marked (figs. 66–72).

From a study of abnormal chick embryos it has been concluded that, although "elevation of the head and proper development of the head fold largely depend on the condition of other structures of the head region," the foregut "develops normally in the absence of the head fold as well as in cases in which the nearby anterior [rostral] end of the neural primordium is defective by malformation or experiment" (Gruenwald, 1941). In other words, the foregut "depends very little upon the condition of the surrounding structures and develops normally whenever there is no mechanical obstacle" (*ibid.*).

The foregut is intimately related dorsally to the floor of the neural groove. At first a shallow pocket (of 0.17 mm in Da 1), the recess soon attains a length of 0.5 mm (in No. 1878). Caudally, the foregut appears triangular or even T-shaped on cross section, and it presents internally a trough in its floor as well as a corresponding ventral keel externally. The keel is closely related to the developing heart, and the trough indicates the general site of the future respiratory groove. In some embryos (Da 1 and Prague No. 2008), however, the keel is scarcely developed and the foregut is oval or reniform (fig. 67) rather than triangular in cross section. The "earliest trace" of the first pharyngeal pouches (fig. 62) and perhaps an "early indication" of the first pharyngeal cleft have been detected in one specimen (Ingalls, 1920).[2]

---

[2] It is now nearly half a century since, in a discussion of "fishy nomenclature," it was proposed that the word "branchial" be dropped from mammalian embryology (Frazer, 1923). The visceral pouches of embryonic reptiles, birds, and mammals "bear little resemblance to the gill-slits of the adult fish" but rather "resemble the visceral pouches which appear in the *embryonic* stages of fish" (de Beer, 1958). Indeed, "all that can be said is that the fish preserves its visceral pouches and elaborates them into its gill-slits, while reptiles, birds, and mammals do not preserve them as such, but convert them into other structures" (*ibid.*). "Gastrula" and "gastrulation" are additional examples of terms that are not properly applicable to mammals (van Oordt, 1921), except, of course, in the very general sense that:

"La gastrulation n'est que mouvements, mais ces mouvements nous les retrouvons identiques chez tous les Chordés. Eux seuls constituent la constante qui nous permettra de définir l'essence même de la gastrulation: la mise en place dans la profondeur du germe de territoires situés d'abord en superficie" (Pasteels, 1940).

STAGE 9

The oropharyngeal (or buccopharyngeal) membrane, absent at first (in Da 1), becomes quite well defined (fig. 63) and attains a width of about 0.05 mm (in No. 1878). The stomodeum is beginning to form.

Although a pit in the ventral wall of the foregut has been claimed to represent the beginning of the thyroid gland (Wilson, 1914; Ingalls, 1920), it is likely that the thyroid primordium does not make its appearance until the following stage. Similarly, an indication of the liver is not found until stage 10.

In the chick embryo, the hindgut has been described as initially a hollowing out of the ventral portion of the "trunk-tail-node" and its "formation is not the result of a folding" of the blastoderm (Gruenwald, 1941).

Primitive streak. The primitive streak extends from the cloacal membrane to the neurenteric canal. Rarely can its entire extent be appreciated in dorsal view (H3); usually it appears foreshortened (No. 1878) and may also be curved (Da 1). A primitive groove may be found but a distinct node may not always be readily distinguishable. When the obliquity and curvature of the streak are taken into account, the primitive streak occupies one-third (Da 1; H3) to one-quarter (No. 5080; No. 1878) of the length of the embryo. This fraction becomes further reduced during stages 10 and 11 (Bartelmez and Evans, 1926).

Mesoderm. The mesoderm, as the mesoblast may perhaps now be termed, is arranged on each side as (a) a longitudinal, paraxial band (nicely shown in Ludwig's reconstruction, plate 2, figs. 3 and 4) and (b) a lateral plate. The paraxial mesoderm is beginning to become segmented in the junctional region between brain and spinal cord. The somites, one to three pairs, may differ in number on the two sides of the body (No. 1878). Cavities (the so-called myocoeles) may be detectable in the somites (fig. 69). The first pair of somites appear just caudal to the midpoint of the notochordal plate (No. 5080).

Although no nephric structures are found until stage 10, the general region of the intermediate mesoderm can be made out in stage 9 between the paraxial mesoderm and the lateral plate. (It is particularly clear, for example, on the right side of sections 115 to 117 of embryo Da 1.)

Coelom. The appearance of the coelom has the effect of splitting the lateral plate into somatopleuric and splanchnopleuric layers.

The pericardial cavity (figs. 60, 65, 67, and 68), which is first seen at the end of stage 8, appears as a horseshoe-shaped space, together with associated vesicles, within the mesoderm of the rostral half of the embryo (No. 5080, Davis, 1927, figs. 2 and 3; Da 1, Ludwig, 1928, fig. 2). The limbs of the horseshoe begin blindly on each side at the level of the first somite. Here the cavities closely approach the extra-embryonic coelom although the intra-embryonic coelom remains closed throughout. At first the right and left limbs do not intercommunicate (No. 5080) but soon do so (Da 1; No. 1878). The small, discrete vesicles associated with the limbs of the horseshoe are coelomic spaces that have not as yet joined the larger cavities. They suggest the mode of coelomic cavity formation, namely, the fusion of discrete vesicles. Some indications of coelomic formation caudally may be detected (Ludwig, 1928) and distinct bilateral cavities are present in one specimen (fig. 71).

Blood vascular system. Blood vessels are arising in several separate regions

(Ingalls, 1920): the chorion, the body stalk, the yolk sac, and the embryo proper, together with its amnion. The connections between these vessels are secondary, and they are established at various times and in a number of different places.

Within the body of the embryo, the two omphalomesenteric veins are distinguishable. Each enters the corresponding horn of the sinus venosus. Also present within the body are the first pair of aortic arches, the beginning of the internal carotid arteries, and, at least in an interrupted course, the two dorsal aortae (Ingalls, 1920). A closed circulation, however, is not yet present. The aortae constitute medial vascular tracts, whereas lateral tracts consist of the vitelline veins and the cardiac rudiments (Ludwig, 1928, plate 3, fig. 6). It seems that the connection of the vitelline plexus with the aorta caudally antedates the connection with the heart rostrally (Ingalls, 1920). In No. 1878 the sole union of intra- and extra-embryonic vessels is provided by the aorta, which communicates (at least unilaterally) with the vitelline plexus. Either no blood cells (Da 1) or a few cells in the aorta (No. 1878) are found within the body of the embryo.

From his study of No. 5080, Davis (1927) concluded that whereas the possibility of an extra-embryonic origin for the cardiac primordium could not definitely be excluded, "it can be stated with certainty that no connection exists between the well-differentiated angioblastic tissue of the yolk-sac and that of the heart." In brief, "the evidence strongly leans toward an intra-embryonic origin, that is, from the cardiogenic plate."

The cardiogenic plate (of Mollier) is the ventral (splanchnic) wall of the pericardial cavity, and from it the epimyocardium (or at least the myocardium) is believed to be derived. The endocardium (fig. 65) is represented at first by a network of mesenchymal cells between the cardiogenic plate and the endoderm. This endocardial plexus, which is at first (Da 1) mostly solid and paired, soon becomes divisible into three parts: atrial, ventricular, and conal (bulbar). The cellular cords that form the plexus become canalized, and their cavities become confluent (Orts Llorca, Jiménez Collado, and Ruano Gil, 1960).

The conoventricular region (see O'Rahilly, 1971, for terminology) occupies the median plane in No. 1878, in which two ventricular roots unite with each other. Rostrally, the cardiac plexus gives way to the first pair of aortic arches, which in turn lead to the dorsal aortae. The atrial components remain bilateral until a subsequent stage. It is possible that the conoventricular part of the heart, rather than being formed by fusion of paired primordia, arises *in situ* from an elaboration of mesoderm bridging the rostral end of the embryonic disc during the presomite phase (Allan, in Ebert, 1963).

With regard to the external appearance of the heart, three sulci have appeared in No. 1878: (a) atrioventricular, (b) interventricular (bulboventricular), and (c) conotruncal (interbulbar; infundibulotruncal). It should be kept in mind, however, that the cardiac region of this embryo appears to be distorted.

Other features that have been identified by stage 9 include the "cardiac jelly" (Davis, 1927), the mesocardium, and the septum transversum (Ingalls, 1920).

Notochordal plate. The notochordal plate (about 0.66 mm in length in Da 1) is intercalated into the endoderm (fig. 60). It extends rostrally almost as far as the oropharyngeal membrane and, caudally, it blends with the primitive node. Extracellular granules in the prechordal plate, notochordal process, primitive streak, and neural plate have been noted in presomite and early somite embryos (Allan, 1963).

Neurenteric canal. The neurenteric canal (fig. 60) may be completely patent (Da 1; H3; see Wilson, 1914, fig. 7), only partly patent (No. 5080), or completely closed (No. 1878). The neurenteric canal appears first during stage 8 (e.g., in Dy, R.S., M'Intyre, Gläveke, Vuill.) and is found in some embryos of stages 9 and 10.

Prechordal plate. The fusion of the rostral end of the notochordal plate with the mesoderm in Da 1 was thought by Hill and Florian (1931b) to be the prechordal plate. It was believed to be identifiable in embryo Gv also.

Yolk sac (fig. 67). Blood islands are numerous and a vitelline plexus is visible. A small yolk sac diverticulum has been described (No. 1878).

Cloacal membrane. Even now, this union of ectoderm and endoderm "is in a way hardly a membrane" (Ingalls, 1920).

Allantoic diverticulum. Either an allanto-enteric (Da 1) or an allantoic (No. 1878) diverticulum may be present. It runs between the umbilical arteries (fig. 62).

In the chick, rotation at the caudal end of the embryo alters the allantois in such a way that it becomes partly unfolded (Gruenwald, 1941). The allantois then becomes a shallow diverticulum of the hindgut (*ibid.*, fig. 6) although "it is highly probable . . . that the proximal part of the allantoic pocket contributes to the formation of the floor of the hindgut."

Connecting stalk. The vascular channels are well developed and occupy most of the stalk, which is quite thick. The right and left umbilical arteries are readily distinguishable, one on each side of the allantoic diverticulum. The future umbilical veins are represented by a vascular plexus which communicates with the arteries. Blood islands have been identified in the connecting stalk as well as over the yolk sac.

SPECIMENS OF STAGE 9 IN CARNEGIE COLLECTION

These are listed in order of serial number in Table 16.

SPECIMENS OF STAGE 9 ALREADY DESCRIBED

(listed in order of number of pairs of somites)

1 somite pair, Carnegie No. 5080. Studied and illustrated by Davis (1927, figs. 2–5 and 39–42) and Severn (1971, figs. 1–4). First pair of somites not separate rostrally and contain no myocoeles (Arey, 1938). Chorion, 14.5 × 1.5 mm. Embryonic disc, 1.5 mm.

1 somite pair. Another specimen, described briefly by Bagiński and Borsuk (1967).

2 somite pairs, Da 1 (Dann). An important specimen (fig. 60) possessing 2 pairs of somites (Studnička, 1929; Florian and Völker, 1929; Arey, 1938), although featured originally as having only one. Described and illustrated in detail by Ludwig (1928). Removed from uterus. Chorion, 12 mm. Embryo, 1.8 mm in a straight line, 2.4 mm by flexible scale. Sectioned transversely at 8 micrometers. Stained with alum cochineal. Neurenteric canal present. Sections are housed in the Anatomisches Institut, Basel. Photographic negatives of sections are filed in Carnegie Collection under No.

TABLE 16. List of Specimens of Stage 9 in Carnegie Collection

Serial No.	Somite Pairs	Size(mm)	Grade	Fixative	Cutting Medium	Plane	Thinness (micrometers)	Stain	Date and Donor	Remarks
1878	2–3	Ch., 12 ×10.5 ×7.5 E., 1.38	Good	Formol	P	Cor.	10	H.-E.	1917, E. J. O'Shaughnessy, New Canaan, Conn.	Described by Ingalls, 1920
5080	1	Ch., 14.5 E., 1.5	Poor	Formol	P	Trans.	10	Al. coch.	1926, S. P. Hoffman, Fort Wayne, Ind.	Studied by Davis, 1927
7650	2–3	E., 2–3	Good	Alc. & Bouin	C-P	Trans.	6	H.-E.	1939, A. T. Hertig, Boston, Mass.	Said to be female (Park, 1957)

STAGE 9

5982. Presumed age, about 21 days. Dorsal and median projections published (*ibid.*, figs. 1 and 2; Florian and Völker, 1929, fig. 14).

2–3 somite pairs, H3. Described by Wilson (1914), according to whom it "possessed probably two, possibly three, pairs of somites." Chorion, 8.5 × 5.7 ×

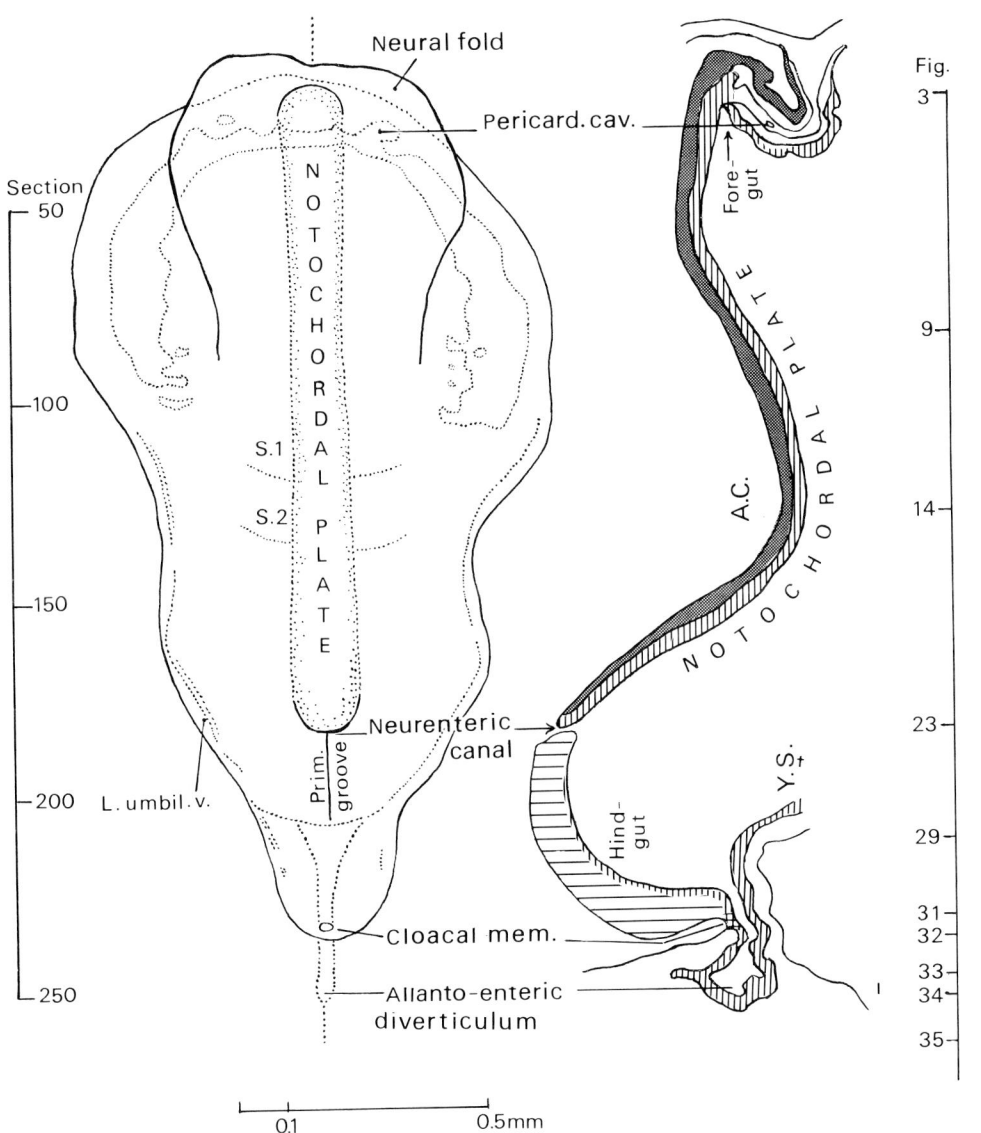

Fig. 60. Dorsal view and median reconstruction of embryo Da 1 (No. 5982), stage 9, in alignment. The dorsal view, which is based on an illustration published by Ludwig (1928, fig. 2), shows the neural folds, pericardial cavity, notochordal plate, and somites. The median reconstruction is based on the same author (his fig. 1). The foregut and hindgut are beginning to form, and the neurenteric canal and the allanto-enteric diverticulum are evident. The figure references are to the sections reproduced by Ludwig among an extensive series of photomicrographs.

5 mm. Embryo, 1.43 mm. Sectioned obliquely (transversely) at 10 micrometers. Stained with hematoxylin. Fixation not adequate for reconstruction. The relatively longer primitive streak suggests that this embryo may be less advanced than No. 1878. Prechordal plate, or at least prechordal mesoderm, figured (Hill and Florian, 1931b). Presumed age, 18–21 days.

2–3 somite pairs, Carnegie No. 1878 (figs. 61–65). An important specimen

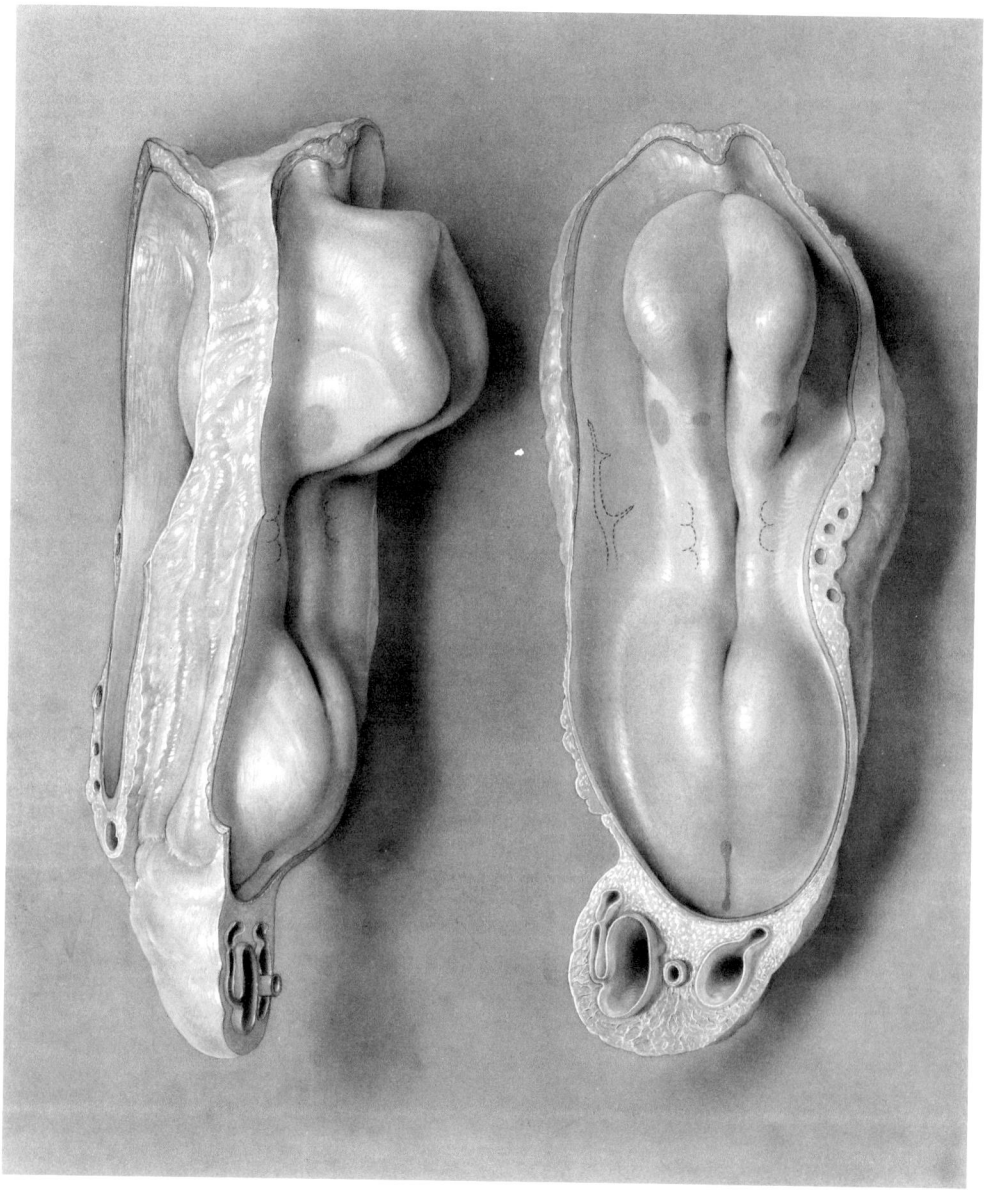

Fig. 61. Left lateral and dorsal views of No. 1878, stage 9, as depicted by Mr. James F. Didusch in 1919. *Cf.* figures 62 and 63. Approximately one-half of the longitudinal extent of the neural groove represents the future brain.

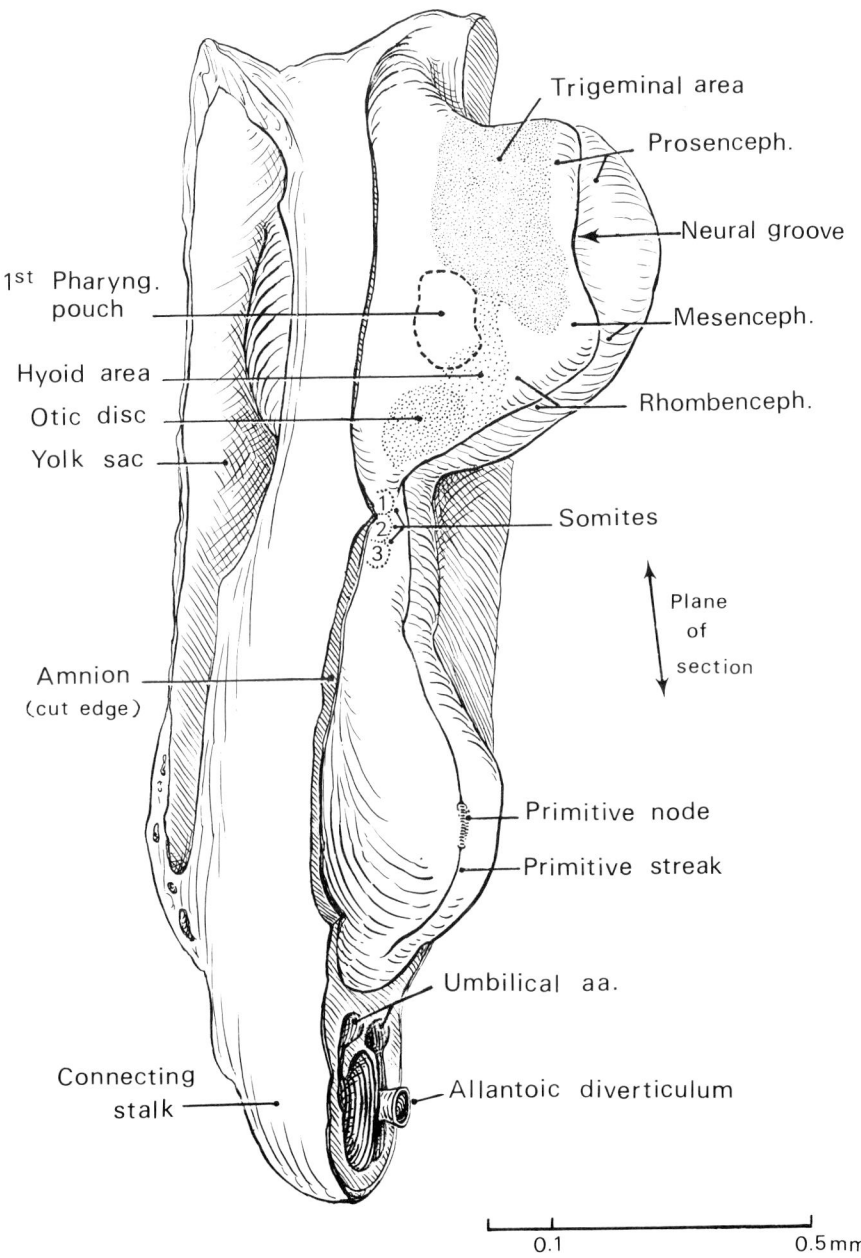

Fig. 62. Left lateral view of No. 1878, stage 9. Based largely on a geometric projection of a reconstruction reproduced by Bartelmez and Evans (1926, Plate 3, fig. 3). The ectodermal areas of the cephalic region are indicated by stippling. The cranial (or mesencephalic) flexure of the brain is evident.

Fig. 63. Dorsal view and median reconstruction of No. 1878, stage 9, in alignment. The dorsal view, which is based on an illustration by Mr. Didusch (see fig. 61), shows the neural folds and groove, the otic discs, and the somites. Medial to the otic discs, areas that possibly represent the trigeminal ganglia are indicated without a label. The median reconstruction is based on an illustration by Mr. Didusch (Ingalls, 1920, Plate 2) and on a drawing reproduced by Bartelmez and Evans (1926, Plate 5, fig. 9). Various features are shown: pericardial cavity, oropharyngeal membrane (O.P.M.), developing pharynx (Phar.), rostral intestinal portal, and allantoic diverticulum.

STAGE 9

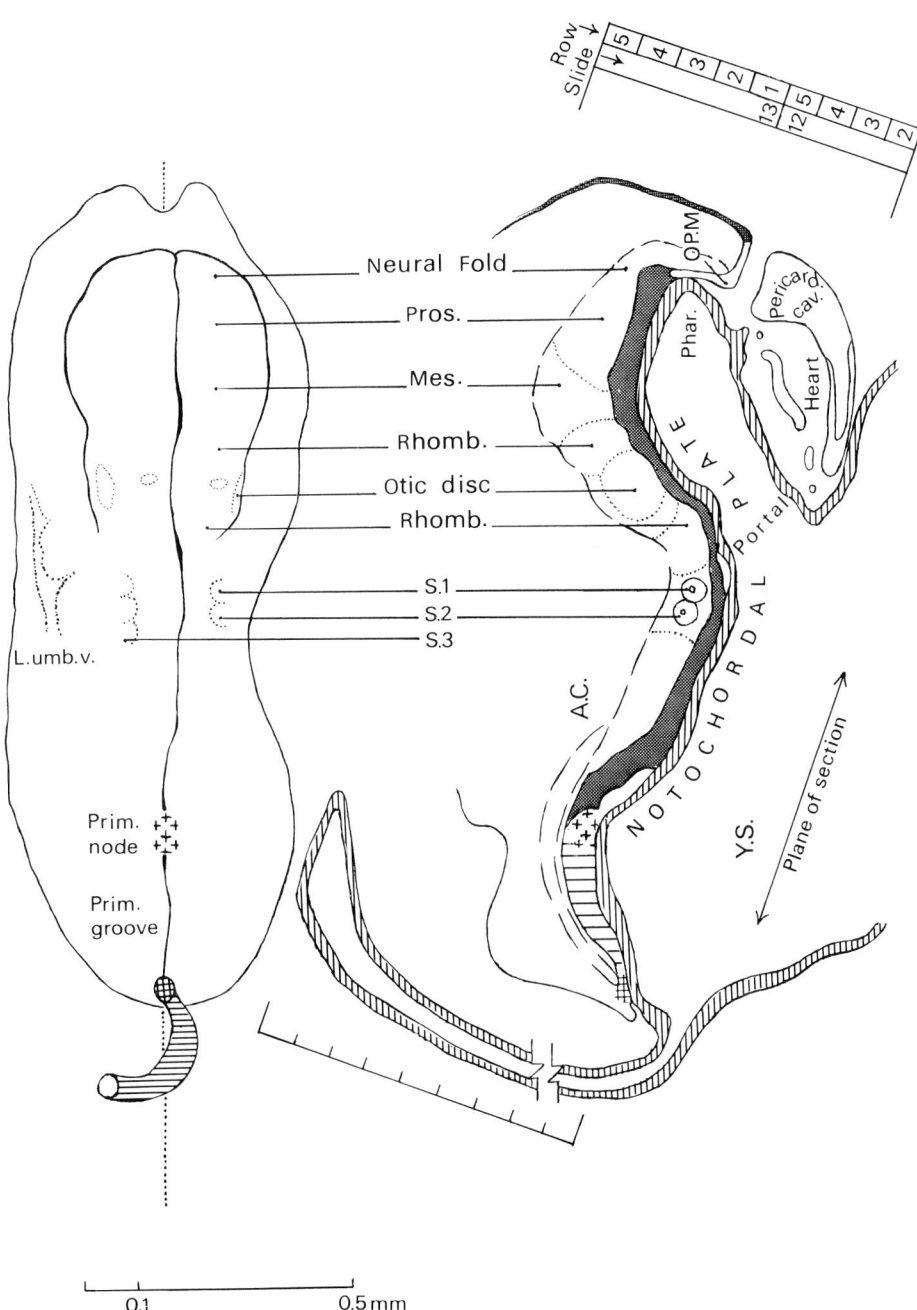

Fig. 64. The neural groove and one of the neural folds of No. 1878, stage 9, in the region of the rhombencephalon. The otic disc is found on the lateral aspect of the neural fold. The basement membrane is visible. The interrupted line (M. P.) indicates the median plane. Section 12-5-7.

Fig. 65. Oblique section through the heart of No. 1878, stage 9. The foregut appears near the upper right-hand corner of the photomicrograph. The U-shaped space is the pericardial cavity. The so-called epimyocardial mantle, the "cardiac jelly," and the endocardial plexus are evident centrally. Section 12-3-5.

STAGE 9

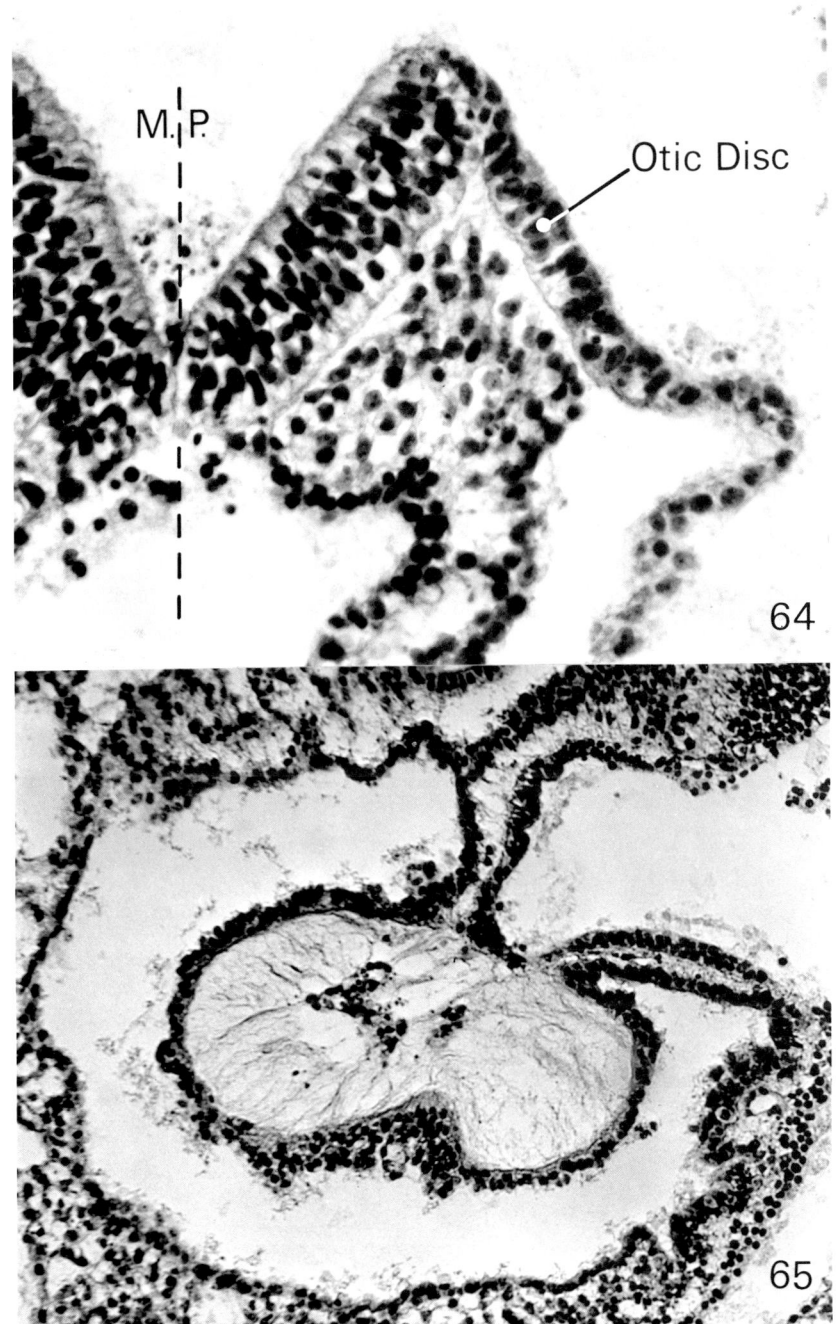

possessing 2 somite pairs on the right side and 3 on the left. Florian (1934b) had certain difficulties and considered the embryo to be too small. Curettage. Chorion, 12 × 10.5 × 7.5 mm. Embryonic disc, 1.38 mm in a straight line. Described in detail and illustrated by Ingalls (1920), who believed that "the earliest recognizable stage of dextrocardia" is present, "to which might have been added later a more or less complete situs inversus viscerum;" at any rate, Davis, (1927), who studied and illustrated the heart, considered that "the cardiac area is distorted." Angiogenesis in chorion described by Hertig (1935). Primitive streak and node, 0.13 mm, according to Ingalls, but about 0.22 mm in fig. 15 of Florian and Völker (1929) and more than 0.3 mm in plate 5, fig. 9, of Bartelmez and Evans (1926). Neurenteric canal not patent but pit present (Bartelmez and Evans, 1926). Median projection published (*ibid.*, plate 5, fig. 9; Florian and Völker, 1929, fig. 15.

3 somite pairs, T439 (Toronto). Possesses 3 pairs of somites (Arey, 1938), although featured originally as having only two. Summarized in an abstract by Piersol (1937). Embryo, 2.03 × 0.72 mm. Sectioned sagittally. Neurenteric canal closed but its remains are evident. Said to contain no blood vessels in any part of the embryo itself.

3 somite pairs, Gv (Madrid). Described by Jiménez Collado and Ruano Gil (1963). Heart described by Orts Llorca, Jiménez Collado, and Ruano Gil (1960). Tubal. Embryo, 1.81 mm. Sectioned at 7 micrometers. Stained with hematoxylin and eosin. Reconstructed. On the basis of its external characters, said to lie between stage 9 and stage 10. Presumed age, 21 ± 1 days.

3 somite pairs, No. 2008 (Prague). Excellent specimen (figs. 66–72) at present being described by Dr. J. E. Jirásek. Embryo, 1.73 mm. Fixed in calcium formol. Sectioned transversely at 10 micrometers. Various stains used, including histochemical procedures.

ADDITIONAL SPECIMEN

The His embryo "E" (2.1 mm) is listed by Bartelmez and Evans (1926) between No. 1878 (2–3 somite pairs) and No. 3709 (4 somite pairs, stage 10).

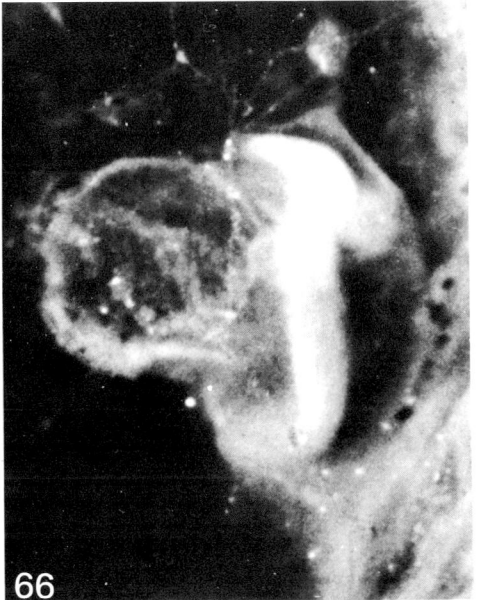

Fig. 66. Left lateral view of Prague embryo No. 2008, stage 9, by courtesy of Dr. J. E. Jirásek. The gentle curvature of the body and the absence of kinking suggest the normal appearance to be expected at this stage. The yolk sac is seen in the left-hand half of the photograph.

Figures 67 to 72 are sections through Prague embryo No. 2008, stage 9, by courtesy of Dr. J. E. Jirásek.

Fig. 67. The amniotic cavity, neural groove, foregut, and yolk sac are evident. The foregut, which appears reniform, has been sectioned immediately rostral to the rostral intestinal portal. The limbs of the pericardial cavity can be seen, one on each side, and the cardiogenic mesoderm is found on the ventral aspect of the cavity.

Fig. 68. A view of the neural groove and pericardioperitoneal canals in the region of the future midgut.

Fig. 69. Transverse section through one of the pairs of somites. So-called myocoeles are visible.

Fig. 70. Section through the hindgut.

Fig. 71. Section through the hindgut and caudally located, bilateral coelomic cavities. The allantoic primordium is visible in cross section in the lowermost portion of the photomicrograph.

Fig. 72. Section through the caudal end of the amniotic cavity (lower quarter of photomicrograph) to show the chorion and the chorionic villi (upper two-thirds of photomicrograph).

STAGE 9

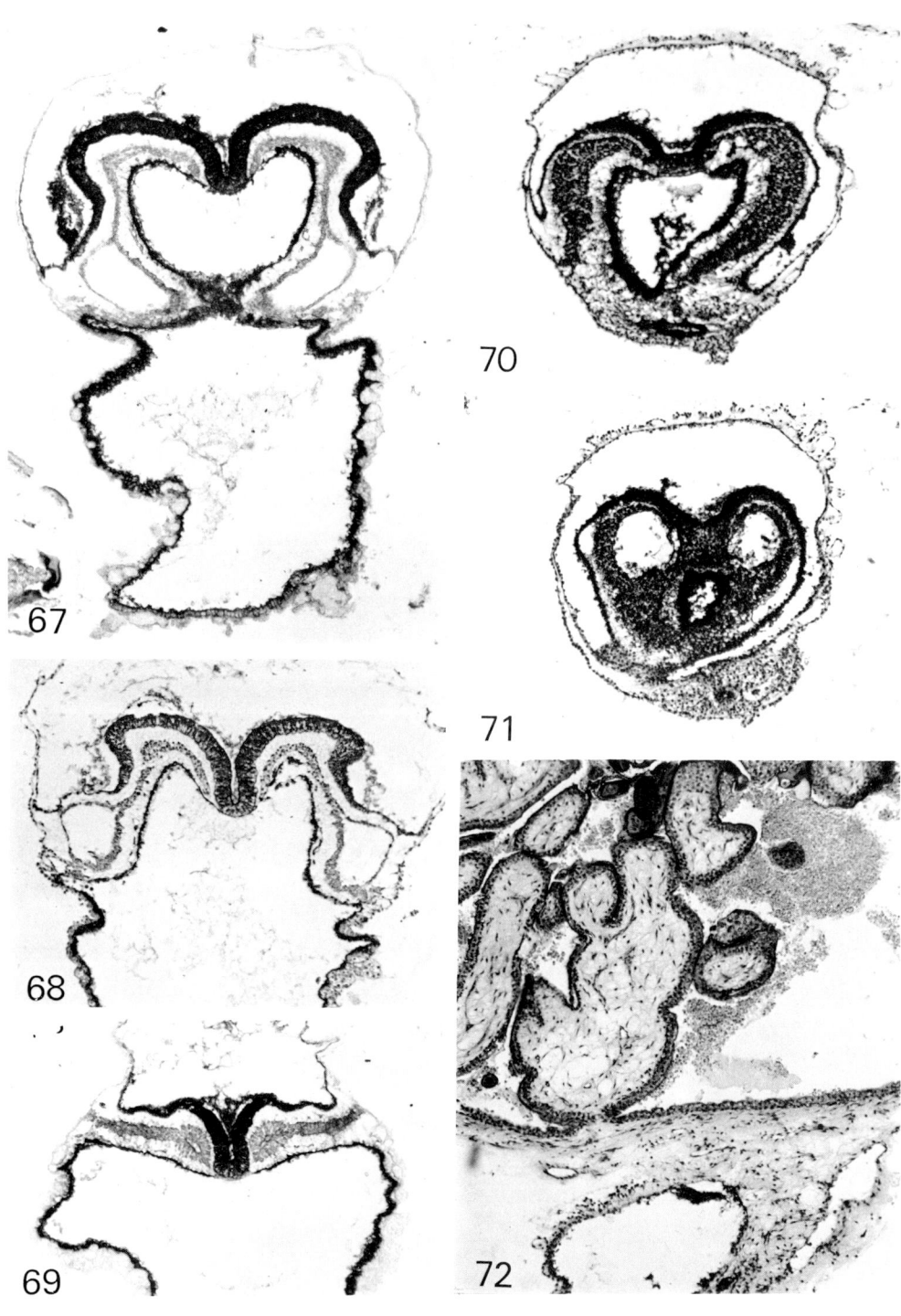

CONCLUDING REMARK

By stage 9, the "embryo proper" has been formed, and an account of the subsequent stages (10 to 23) has already been made available (Heuser and Corner, 1957; Streeter, 1942–1951) although it is now undergoing revision. All 23 stages have been listed in Table 1 and, in conclusion, some summarizing graphs are provided. Figures 74 and 75 present embryonic length from stage 5 to stage 23, and the maximum diameter of the chorion is included in figure 75. In figure 73, the relative sizes of the embryo and the chorion at weekly intervals are shown.

144   EMBRYOS OF THE FIRST THREE WEEKS

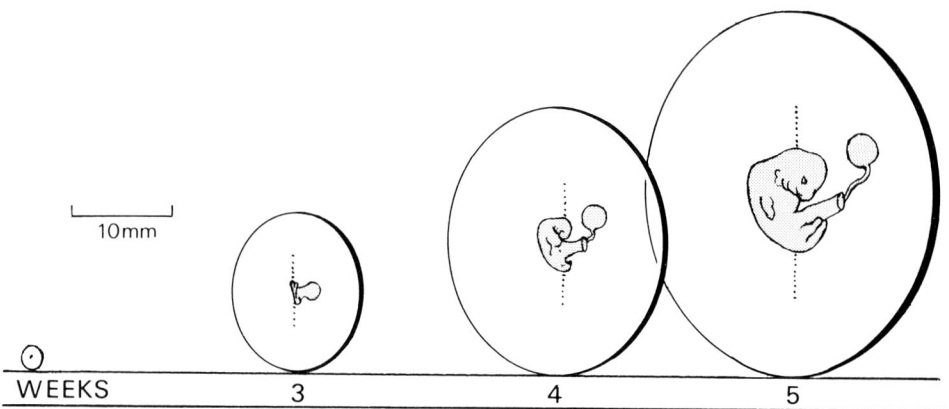

Fig. 73. The relative size of the embryo and the chorion at weekly intervals. The stages shown are 6, 10, 13, 16, 17, 20, and 23. The drawings are 1.4 times greater than the actual size of the specimens.

CONCLUDING REMARK

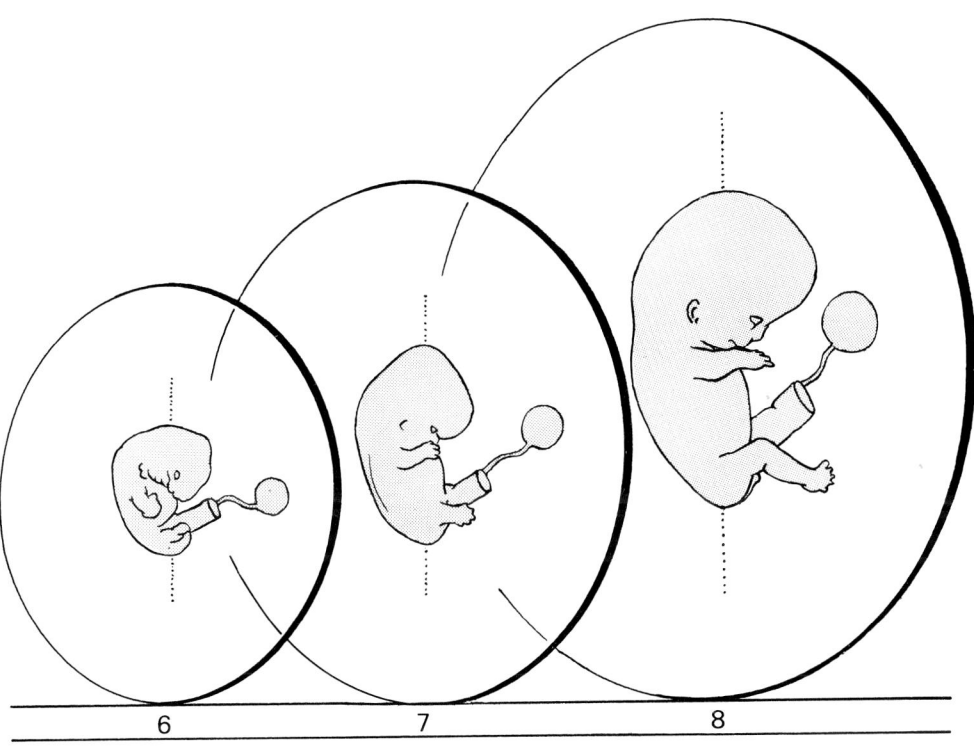

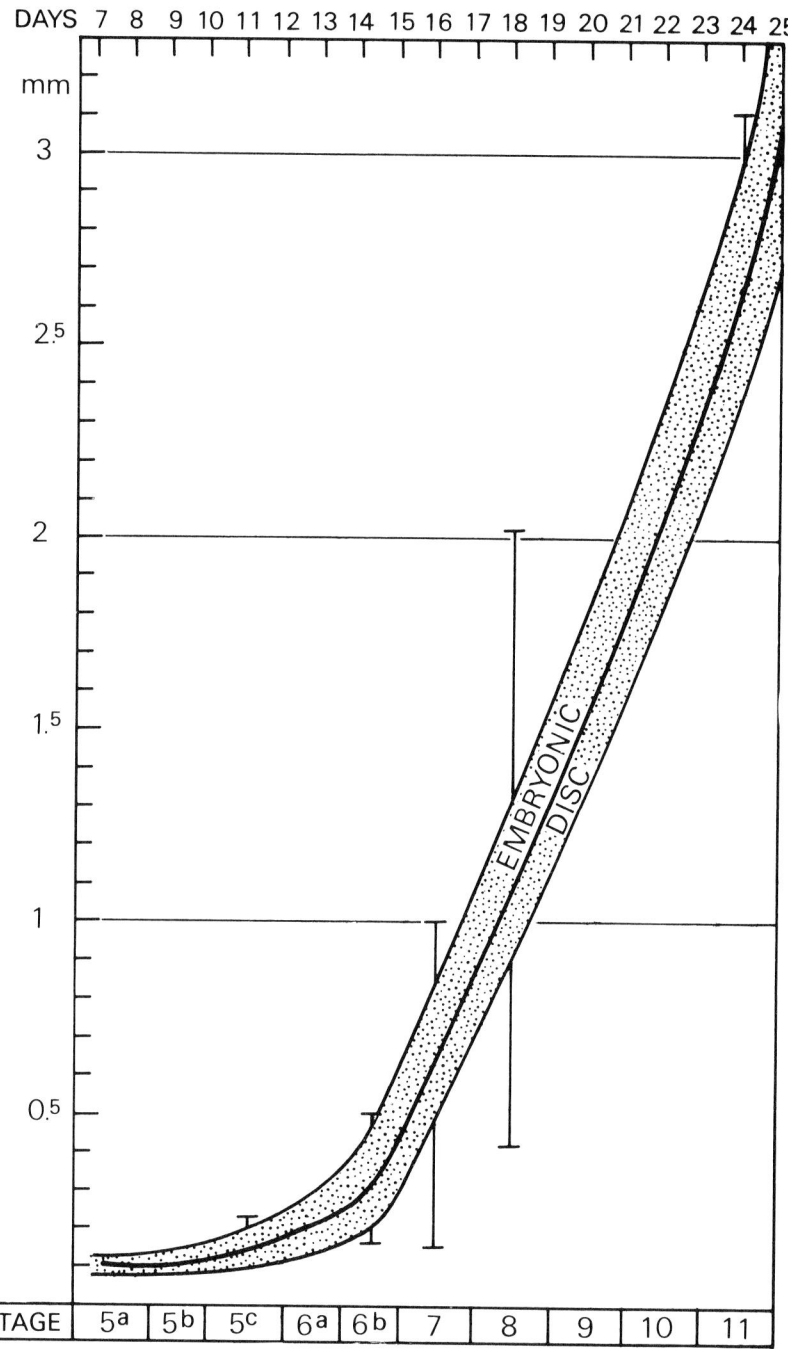

Fig. 74. The length of the embryonic disc from stage 5 to stage 11, approximately 1 to 3½ postovulatory weeks. Based on the measurements of 81 embryos. Most of the specimens may be expected to fall within the shaded band, but extreme values are indicated by the five vertical lines. At 1 week the diameter of the disc is approximately 0.1 mm. At 2 weeks the disc is about 0.2 mm in length. At 3 weeks the embryonic length has increased to about 1.5–2 mm. The measurements at later stages are shown in figure 75.

CONCLUDING REMARK

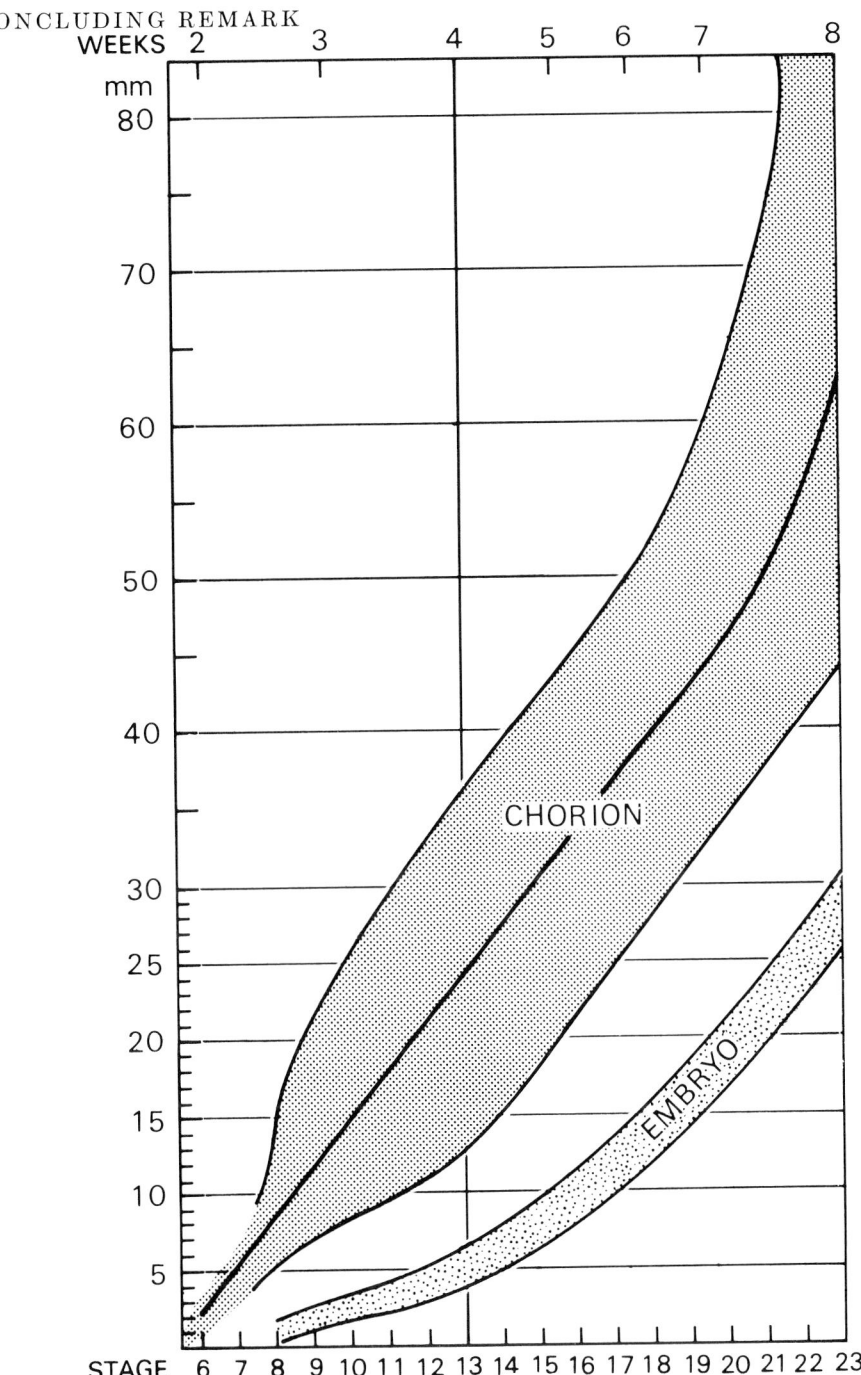

Fig. 75. The length of the embryo from stage 8 to stage 23, approximately 2½ to 8 postovulatory weeks. Based on the measurements of 104 specimens that had been graded as excellent in quality. The C.-R. length has been used in the case of the later stages. The measurements at earlier stages are shown in figure 74. The maximum diameter of the chorion has also been included (based on 185 specimens graded as either good or excellent): the shaded band includes 81 per cent of the specimens. A vertical line is placed at 4 weeks, when the embryo is about 5 mm in length and the chorion about 25 mm in diameter. At 8 weeks, the embryo is about 30 mm in C.-R. length and the chorion is about 65 mm in diameter.

REFERENCES

Aasar, Y. H. 1931. The history of the prochordal plate in the rabbit. *J. Anat.*, London, *46*, 14–45.

Adams, W. E. 1960. Early human development. *N. Z. Med. J., 59*, 7–17.

Adelmann, H. B. 1922. The significance of the prechordal plate: an interpretative study. *Amer. J. Anat., 31*, 54–101.

Allan, F. D. 1963. Observations on the organizer areas of the human pre-somite embryo. *Anat. Rec., 145*, 199.

Allen, E., Pratt, J. P., Newell, Q. U., and Bland, L. J. 1930a. Human ova from large follicles; including a search for maturation divisions and observations on atresia. *Amer. J. Anat., 46*, 1–53.

Allen, E., Pratt, J. P., Newell, Q. U., and Bland, L. J. 1930b. Human tubal ova; related early corpora lutea and uterine tubes. *Carnegie Inst. Wash. Publ. 414, Contrib. Embryol., 22*, 45–76.

Allen, M. S., and Turner, U. G. 1971. Twin birth—identical or fraternal twins? *Obstet. Gynecol., 37*, 538–542.

Arey, L. B. 1938. The history of the first somite. *Carnegie Inst. Wash. Publ. 496, Contrib. Embryol., 27*, 233–269.

D'Arrigo, S. 1961. Illustrazione di un embrione umano al principio della terza settimana di sviluppo. *Riv. Patol. Clin. Sper., 2*, 1–15.

Ashley, D. J. B. 1959. Are ovarian pregnancies parthenogenetic? *Amer. J. Hum. Genet., 11*, 305–310.

Baca, M., and Zamboni, L. 1967. The fine structure of human follicular oocytes. *J. Ultrastruct. Res., 19*, 354–381.

Bagiński, S., and Borsuk, I. 1967. (Micromorphology of the human fetus in the third week of tubal pregnancy). *Folia Morphol.* (Warszawa), *26*, 153–160.

Bandler. 1912. The earliest recorded case of ectopic gestation. *Amer. J. Obstet. Gynecol., 66*, 454.

Bartelmez. G. W., and Evans, H. M. 1926. Development of the human embryo during the period of somite formation, including embryos with 2 to 16 pairs of somites. *Carnegie Inst. Wash. Publ. 362, Contrib. Embryol., 17*, 1–67.

deBeer, G. 1958. *Embryos and Ancestors*. 3rd edition, Clarendon Press, Oxford.

Benoit, J. 1969. Irradiation *in vitro* de la région du noeud de Hensen de la gastrula de souris. *C. R. Acad. Sci. Paris, 269*, 724–727.

Blandau, R. J. (ed.). 1971. *The Biology of the Blastocyst*. University of Chicago Press, Chicago.

Blechschmidt, E. 1968. *Vom Ei zum Embryo*. Deutsche Verlags-Anstalt, Stuttgart.

Blechschmidt, E. 1972. Die ersten drei Wochen nach der Befruchtung. *Image Roche*, Basel, *47*, 17–24.

Bloom, W., and Bartelmez, G. W. 1940. Hematopoiesis in young human embryos. *Amer. J. Anat., 67*, 21–53.

Boerner-Patzelt, D., and Schwarzacher, W. 1923. Ein junges menschliches Ei in situ. *Z. Anat. Entwicklungsgesch., 68,* 204–229.

Born, G. 1883. Die Plattenmodellirmethode. *Arch. Mikr. Anat., 22*, 584–599.

Bourne, G. 1962. *The Human Amnion and Chorion*. Lloyd-Luke, London.

Böving, B. G. 1963. Implantation Mechanisms. Ch. 7 in C. G. Hartman (ed.), *Conference on Physiological Mechanisms Concerned with Conception*. Pergamon, Oxford.

Böving, B. G. 1965. Anatomy of Reproduction. Ch. 1 in J. P. Greenhill, *Obstetrics*. 13th edition, Saunders, Philadelphia.

Bowman, P., and McLaren, A. 1970. Cleavage rate of mouse embryos *in vivo* and *in vitro*. *J. Embryol. Exp. Morphol., 24*, 203–207.

Boyd, J. D., and Hamilton, W. J. 1966. Electron microscopic observations on the cytotrophoblast contribution to the syncytium in the human placenta. *J. Anat.*, London, *100*, 535–548.

Boyd, J. D., and Hamilton, W. J. 1970. *The Human Placenta*. Heffer, Cambridge.

Boyden, E. A. 1955. *A Laboratory Atlas of the 13-mm. Pig Embryo*. Wistar Institute, Philadelphia, 3rd edition.

Brackett, B. G., Seitz, H. M., Rocha, G., and Mastroianni, L. 1972. The mammalian fertilization process. *In* Moghissi, K. S., and Hafez, E. S. E. (ed.). *Biology of Mammalian Fertilization and Implantation*. Thomas, Springfield, Illinois. Ch. 6 (pp 165–184).

Bremer, J. L. 1914. The earliest blood-vessels in man. *Amer. J. Anat., 16*, 447–475.

Brewer, J. I. 1937. A normal human ovum in a stage preceding the primitive streak (The Edwards-Jones-Brewer ovum). *Amer. J. Anat., 61*, 429–481.

Brewer, J. I. 1938. A human embryo in the bilaminar blastodisc stage (The Edwards-Jones-Brewer ovum). *Carnegie Inst. Wash. Publ. 496, Contrib. Embryol.*, 27, 85–93.

Brewer, J. I., and Fitzgerald, J. E. 1937. Six normal and complete presomite human ova. *Amer. J. Obstet. Gynecol.*, 34, 210–224.

Broman, I. 1936. Ein frühembryonales (etwa 20 Tage altes) menschliches Monstrum. *Morphol. Jahrb.*, 78, 421–444.

Bryce, T. H. 1924. Observations on the early development of the human embryo. *Trans. Roy. Soc. Edinburgh*, 53, 533–567.

Bulmer, M. G. 1970. *The Biology of Twinning in Man*. Clarendon Press, Oxford.

Calarco, P. G., and Brown, E. H. 1969. An ultrastructural and cytological study of pre-implantation development of the mouse. *J. Exp. Zool.*, 171, 253–283.

Corner, G. W. 1951. Preface to *Developmental Horizons in Human Embryos: Age Groups XI to XXIII*, by G. L. Streeter. Embryology Reprint, Volume 2. Carnegie Institution of Washington, pp. iii–iv.

Corner, G. W. 1955. The observed embryology of human single-ovum twins and other multiple births. *Amer. J. Obstet. Gynecol.*, 70, 933–951.

Daniel, J. C., and Olson, J. D. 1966. Cell movement, proliferation and death in the formation of the embryonic axis of the rabbit. *Anat. Rec.*, 156, 123–127.

Dankmeijer, J., and Wielenga, G. 1968. Observation d'un oeuf humain d'environ dix jours. *Bull. Ass. Anat.*, 53, 793–796.

Davies, F. 1944. A previllous human ovum, aged nine to ten days (the Davies-Harding ovum). *Trans. Roy. Soc. Edinburgh*, 61, 315–326.

Davis, C. L. 1927. Development of the human heart from its first appearance to the stage found in embryos of twenty paired somites. *Carnegie Inst. Wash. Publ. 380, Contrib. Embryol.*, 19, 245–284.

Debeyre, A. 1912. Description d'un embryon humain de 0 mm. 9. *J. Anat. Physiol.*, Paris, 48, 448–515.

Debeyre, A. 1933. Sur la présence de gonocytes chez un embryon humain au stade de la ligne primitive. *C. R. Ass. Anat.*, 28, 240–250.

Dedek, J. F. 1972. *Human Life. Some Moral Issues*. Sheed and Ward, New York.

Dible, J. H., and West, C. M. 1941. A human ovum at the previllous stage. *J. Anat.*, London, 75, 269–281.

Dickmann, Z., Chewe [Clewe], T. H., Bonney, W. A., and Noyes, R. W. 1965. The human egg in the pronuclear stage. *Anat. Rec.*, 152, 293–302.

Dickson, A. D. 1966. The form of the mouse blastocyst. *J. Anat.*, London, 100, 335–348.

Doyle, L. L., Lippes, J., Winters, H. S., and Margolis, A. J. 1966. Human ova in the fallopian tube. *Amer. J. Obstet. Gynecol.*, 95, 115–117.

Edwards, R. G. 1972. Fertilization and cleavage *in vitro* of human ova. In Moghissi, K. S., and Hafez, E. S. E. (ed.). *Biology of Mammalian Fertilization and Implantation*. Thomas, Springfield, Illinois. Ch. 9 (pp 263–278).

Edwards, R. G., Bavister, B. D., and Steptoe, P. C. 1969. Early stages of fertilization *in vitro* of human oocytes matured *in vitro*. *Nature*, 221, 632–635.

Edwards, R. G., Donahue, R. P., Baranki, T. A., and Jones, H. W. 1966. Preliminary attempts to fertilize human oocytes matured in vitro. *Amer. J. Obstet. Gynecol.*, 96, 192–200.

Edwards, R. G., and Fowler, R. E. 1970. Human embryos in the laboratory. *Sci. Amer.*, 223, 44–54.

Edwards, R. G., Steptoe, P. C., and Purdy, J. M. 1970. Fertilization and cleavage *in vitro* of preovulator[y] human oocytes *Nature*, 227, 1307–1309.

Enders, A. C. 1965. Formation of syncytium from cytotrophoblast in the human placenta. *Obstet. Gynecol.*, 25, 378–386.

Enders, A. C., and Schlafke, S. 1967. A morphological analysis of the early implantation stages in the rat. *Amer. J. Anat.*, 120, 185–225.

Eternod, A. C. F. 1899a. Premiers stades de la circulation sanguine dans l'oeuf et l'embryon humains. *Anat. Anz.*, 15, 181–189.

Eternod, A. C. F. 1899b. Il y a un canal notochordal dans l'embryon humain. *Anat. Anz.*, 16, 131–143.

Eternod, A. C. F. 1909. *L'oeuf humain*. Georg, Geneva.

Faber, V. 1940. Beobachtungen an einem etwa 2 Wochen alten menschlichen Ei. *Z. Mikrosk.-Anat. Forsch.*, 48, 375–386.

Fahrenholz, C. 1927. Ein junges menschliches Abortivei. *Z. Mikrosk.-Anat. Forsch.*, 8, 250–324.

Fetzer, M. 1910. Über ein durch Operation gewonnenes menschliches Ei, das in seiner Entwickelung etwa dem Petersschen Ei entspricht. *Verh. Anat. Ges., Erg. Heft. Anat. Anz.*, 37, 116–126.

REFERENCES

Fetzer, M., and Florian, J. 1929. Der jüngste menschliche Embryo (Embryo "Fetzer") mit bereits entwickelter Kloakenmembran. *Anat. Anz.*, 67, 481–492.

Fetzer, M., and Florian, J. 1930. Der Embryo "Fetzer" mit beginnender Axialmesodermbildung und bereits angelegter Kloakenmembran. *Z. Mikrosk.-Anat. Forsch.*, 21, 351–461.

Florian, J. 1927. Über zwei junge menschliche Embryonen. *Verh. Anat. Ges., Erg. Heft Anat. Anz.*, 63, 184–192.

Florian, J. 1928a. Ein junges menschliches Ei in situ (Embryo T. F. mit Primitivstreifen ohne Kopffortsatz). *Z. Mikrosk.-Anat. Forsch.*, 13, 500–590.

Florian, J. 1928b. Grafická rekonstrukce velmi mladých lidských zárodků (Graphische Rekonstruktion sehr junger menschlicher Embryonen). *Spisy Lékařské Fakulty Masarykovy University v Brně*, ČSR (Publications de la Faculté de Médecine, Brno, Répub. Tchécosl.), 6, 1–64.

Florian, J. 1930. The formation of the connecting stalk and the extension of the amniotic cavity towards the tissue of the connecting stalk in young human embryos. *J. Anat.*, London, 64, 454–476.

Florian, J. 1931. "Urkeimzellen" bei einem 625 μ langen menschlichen Embryo. *Verh. Anat. Ges., Erg. Heft Anat. Anz.*, 72, 286.

Florian, J. 1933. The early development of man, with special reference to the development of the mesoderm and the cloacal membrane. *J. Anat.*, London, 67, 263–276.

Florian, J. 1934a. Über die Existenz von zwei verschiedenen Typen junger menschlicher Embryonen. *Biol. Gen.*, 10, 521–532.

Florian, J. 1934b. Ein Schema der Entwicklung der Axialgebilde des menschlichen Embryos bis in das Stadium von 10 Urwirbelpaaren. *Biol. Gen.*, 10, 533–544.

Florian, J. 1934c. Über einige bisher unkorrigiert gebliebene fehlerhafte Angaben der junge menschliche Embryonen beschreibenden Arbeiten. *Anat. Anz.*, 78, 445–450.

Florian, J. 1945. Gastrulace a notogenese obratlovců, zuláště člověka (La gastrulation et la notogénèse des vertébrés, surtout de l'homme). *Věstník Královské České Společnosti Nauk Třída Matematicko-Přírodovědecká*, Ročník, 1–26.

Florian, J., and Beneke, R. 1931. Neue Befunde am Embryo "Beneke." *Verh. Anat. Ges., Erg. Heft Anat. Anz.*, 71, 229–232.

Florian, J., and Hill, J. P. 1935. An early human embryo (No. 1285, Manchester Collection), with capsular attachment of the connecting stalk. *J. Anat.*, London, 69, 399–411.

Florian, J., and Völker, O. 1929. Über die Entwicklung des Primitivstreifens, der Kloakenmembran und der Allantois beim Menschen. *Z. Mikrosk.-Anat. Forsch.*, 16, 75–100.

Fraser, R. C. 1954. Studies on the hypoblast of the young chick embryo. *J. Exp. Zool.*, 126, 349–399.

Frassi, L. 1908. Weitere Ergebnisse des Studiums eines jungen menschlichen Eies in situ. *Arch. Mikr. Anat. Entwicklungsgesch.*, 71, 667–695.

Frazer, J. E. 1923. The nomenclature of diseased states caused by certain vestigial structures in the neck. *Brit. J. Surg.*, 11, 131–136.

Fruhling, L., Ginglinger, A., and Gandar, R. 1954. Oeuf humain âgé de 8 jours. *Bull. Féd. Gynécol. Obstét. Franç.*, 6, 110–111.

Gaunt, W. A. 1971. *Microreconstruction*. Pitman, London.

Gedda, L. 1961. *Twins in History and Science*. Thomas, Springfield, Illinois.

George, W. C. 1942. A presomite human embryo with chorda canal and prochordal plate. *Carnegie Inst. Wash. Publ.* 541, *Contrib. Embryol.*, 30, 1–7.

Giacomini, C. 1898. Un oeuf humain de 11 jours. *Arch. Ital. Biol.*, 29, 1–22.

Gilbert, P. W. 1957. The origin and development of the human extrinsic ocular muscles. *Carnegie Inst. Wash. Publ.* 611, *Contrib. Embryol.*, 36, 59–78.

Gilmour, J. R. 1941. Normal haemopoiesis in intra-uterine and neonatal life. *J. Pathol. Bacteriol.*, 52, 25–55.

Gladstone, R. J., and Hamilton, W. J. 1941. A presomite human embryo (Shaw) with primitive streak and chorda canal, with special reference to the development of the vascular system. *J. Anat.*, London, 76, 9–44.

Greenhill, J. P. 1927. A young human ovum in situ. *Amer. J. Anat.*, 40, 315–354.

Grosser, O. 1913. Ein menschlicher Embryo mit Chordakanal. *Anat. Hefte*, 47, 649–686.

Grosser, O. 1922. Zur Kenntnis der Trophoblastschale bei jungen menschlichen Eiern. *Z. Anat. Entwicklungsgesch.*, 66, 179–198.

Grosser, O. 1926. Trophoblastschwache und zottenarme menschliche Eier. *Z. Mikrosk.-Anat. Forsch.*, 5, 197–220.

Grosser, O. 1931a. Primitivstreifen und Kopffortsatz beim Menschen. *Verh. Anat. Ges., Erg. Heft Anat. Anz.*, 71, 135–139.

Grosser, O. 1931b. Der Kopffortsatz des Primitivstreifens beim Menschen. Seine Differenzierung bei dem Embryo Wa 17. *Z. Anat. Entwicklungsgesch.*, 94, 275–292.

Grosser, O. 1931c. Weiteres über den Primitivstreifen des Menschen. *Verh. Anat. Ges., Erg. Heft Anat. Anz., 72,* 42–44.

Gruenwald, P. 1941. Normal and abnormal detachment of body and gut from the blastoderm in the chick embryo, with remarks on the early development of the allantois. *J. Morphol., 69,* 83–125.

Hadek, R. 1969. *Mammalian Fertilization. An Atlas of Ultrastructure.* Academic Press, New York.

Häggström, P. 1922. Über degenerative "parthenogenetische" Teilungen von Eizellen in normalen Ovarien des Menschen. *Acta Gynecol. Scand., 1,* 137–168.

Hamburger, V., and Hamilton, H. L. 1951. A series of normal stages in the development of the chick embryo. *J. Morphol., 88,* 49–92.

Hamilton, W. J. 1944. Phases of maturation and fertilization in human ova. *J. Anat.,* London, *78,* 1–4.

Hamilton, W. J. 1946. The first findings of a pronuclear stage in man. *J. Anat.,* London, *80,* 224.

Hamilton, W. J. 1949. Early stages of human development. *Ann. R. Coll. Surg. Engl., 4,* 281–294.

Hamilton, W. J., Barnes, J., and Dodds, G. H. 1943. Phases of maturation, fertilization and early development in man. *J. Obstet. Gynaecol., Brit. Emp., 50,* 241–245.

Hamilton, W. J., and Boyd, J. D. 1950. Phases of human development. Ch. 8 in K. Bowes (ed.), *Modern Trends in Obstetrics and Gynaecology.* Butterworth, London, pp. 114–137.

Hamilton, W. J., and Boyd, J. D. 1960. Development of the human placenta in the first three months of gestation. *J. Anat.,* London, *94,* 297–328.

Hamilton, W. J., Boyd, J. D., and Misch, K. A. 1967. A very early monozygotic abnormal twin pregnancy. *Proc. Roy. Soc. Med., 60,* 995–998.

Hamilton, W. J., and Gladstone, R. J. 1942. A presomite human embryo (Shaw): the implantation. *J. Anat.,* London, *76,* 187–203.

Hamilton, W. J., and Laing, J. A. 1946. Development of the egg of the cow up to the stage of blastocyst formation. *J. Anat.,* London, *80,* 194–204.

Hamilton, W. J., and Samuel, D. M. 1956. The early development of the golden hamster (*Cricetus auratus*). *J. Anat.,* London, *90,* 395–416.

Harris, J. W. S., and Ramsey, E. M. 1966. The morphology of human uteroplacental vasculature. *Carnegie Inst. Wash. Publ. 625, Contrib. Embryol., 38,* 43–58.

Harrison, R. G. See Wilens (1969).

Harrison, R. G., and Jeffcoate, T. N. A. 1953. A presomite human embryo showing an early stage of the primitive streak. *J. Anat.,* London, *87,* 124–129.

Harrison, R. G., Jones, C. H., and Jones, E. P. 1966. A pathological presomite human embryo. *J. Pathol. Bacteriol., 92,* 583–584.

Heard, O. O. 1957. Methods used by C. H. Heuser in preparing and sectioning early embryos. *Carnegie Inst. Wash. Publ. 611, Contrib. Embryol., 36,* 1–18.

Heine, Dr., and Hofbauer, J. 1911. Beitrag zur frühesten Eientwicklung. *Z. Geburtsh. Gynäkol., 68,* 665–688.

Hendrickx, A. G. 1971. *Embryology of the Baboon.* University of Chicago Press, Chicago.

Herranz, G., and Vázquez, J. J. 1964. Partenogénesis rudimentaria en el óvulo humano. *Rev. Med. Univ. Navarra, 8,* 115–120.

Hertig, A. T. 1935. Angiogenesis in the early human chorion and in the primary placenta of the macaque monkey. *Carnegie Inst. Wash. Publ. 459, Contrib. Embryol., 25,* 37–81.

Hertig, A. T. 1968. *Human Trophoblast.* Thomas, Springfield, Ill.

Hertig, A. T., Adams, E. C., McKay, D. G., Rock, J., Mulligan, W. J., and Menkin, M. F. 1958. A thirteen-day human ovum studied histochemically. *Amer. J. Obstet. Gynecol., 76,* 1025–1043.

Hertig, A. T., and Rock, J. 1941. Two human ova of the pre-villous stage, having an ovulation age of about eleven and twelve days respectively. *Carnegie Inst. Wash. Publ. 525, Contrib. Embryol., 29,* 127–156.

Hertig, A. T., and Rock, J. 1944. On the development of the early human ovum, with special reference to the trophoblast of the previllous stage: a description of 7 normal and 5 pathologic human ova. *Amer. J. Obstet. Gynecol., 47,* 149–184.

Hertig, A. T., and Rock, J. 1945a. Two human ova of the pre-villous stage, having a developmental age of about seven and nine days respectively. *Carnegie Inst. Wash. Publ. 557, Contrib. Embryol., 31,* 65–84.

Hertig, A. T., and Rock, J. 1945b. On a normal human ovum not over 7½ days of age. *Anat. Rec., 91,* 281.

Hertig, A. T., and Rock, J. 1945c. On a normal ovum of approximately 9 to 10 days of age. *Anat. Rec., 91,* 281.

Hertig, A. T., and Rock, J. 1949. Two human ova of the pre-villous stage, having a developmental age of about eight and nine days respectively. *Carnegie Inst. Wash. Publ. 583, Contrib. Embryol., 33,* 169–186.

REFERENCES

Hertig, A. T., Rock, J., and Adams, E. C. 1956. A description of 34 human ova within the first 17 days of development. *Amer. J. Anat., 98,* 435–493.

Hertig, A. T., Rock, J., Adams, E. C., and Mulligan, W. J. 1954. On the preimplantation stages of the human ovum: a description of four normal and four abnormal specimens ranging from the second to the fifth day of development. *Carnegie Inst. Wash. Publ. 603, Contrib. Embryol., 35,* 199–220.

Herzog, M. 1909. A contribution to our knowledge of the earliest known stages of placentation and embryonic development in man. *Amer. J. Anat., 9,* 361–400.

Hesseldahl, H., and Larsen, J. F. 1969. Ultrastructure of human yolk sac: endoderm, mesenchyme, tubules and mesothelium. *Amer. J. Anat., 126,* 315–335.

van Heukelom, S. 1898. Ueber die menschliche Placentation. *Arch. Anat. Physiol.,* Anat. Abth., 1–35.

Heuser, C. H. 1932a. An intrachorionic mesothelial membrane in young stages of the monkey (Macacus rhesus). *Anat. Rec., 52,* Suppl., 15–16.

Heuser, C. H. 1932b. A presomite human embryo with a definite chorda canal. *Carnegie Inst. Wash. Publ. 433, Contrib. Embryol., 23,* 251–267.

Heuser, C. H. 1954. Monozygotic twin human embryos with an estimated ovulation age of 17 days. *Anat. Rec., 118,* 310.

Heuser, C. H. 1956. A human ovum with an estimated ovulation age of about nine days. *Anat. Rec., 124,* 459.

Heuser, C. H., and Corner, G. W. 1957. Developmental horizons in human embryos. Description of age group X, 4 to 12 somites. *Carnegie Inst. Wash. Publ. 611, Contrib. Embryol., 36,* 29–39.

Heuser, C. H., Rock, J., and Hertig, A. T. 1945. Two human embryos showing early stages of the definitive yolk sac. *Carnegie Inst. Wash. Publ. 557, Contrib. Embryol., 31,* 85–99.

Heuser, C. H., and Streeter, G. L. 1929. Early stages in the development of pig embryos, from the period of initial cleavage to the time of the appearance of limb-buds. *Carnegie Inst. Wash. Publ. 394, Contrib. Embryol., 20,* 1–29.

Heuser, C. H., and Streeter, G. L. 1941. Development of the macaque embryo. *Carnegie Inst. Wash. Publ. 525, Contrib. Embryol., 29,* 15–55.

Hill, J. P. 1932. The developmental history of the Primates. *Phil. Trans. Roy. Soc. London* B, *221,* 45–178.

Hill, J. P., and Florian, J. 1931a. The development of head-process and prochordal plate in man. *J. Anat.,* London, *45,* 242–246.

Hill, J. P., and Florian, J. 1931b. A young human embryo (embryo Dobbin) with head-process and prochordal plate. *Phil. Trans. Roy. Soc. London* B, *219,* 443–486.

Hill, J. P., and Florian, J. 1931c. Further note on the prochordal plate in man. *J. Anat.,* London, *46,* 46–47.

Hill, J. P., and Florian, J. 1963. The development of the primitive streak, head-process and annular zone in *Tarsius,* with comparative notes on *Loris. Bibliog. Primatol., 2,* 1–90.

Hill, J. P., and Tribe, M. 1924. The early development of the cat (Felis domestica). *Quart. J. Microsc. Sci., 68,* 513–602.

Hillman, N., and Tasca, R. J. 1969. Ultrastructural and autoradiographic studies of mouse cleavage stages. *Amer. J. Anat., 126,* 151–173.

Hiramatsu, K. 1936. Ein junges Menschenei (Ei-Andô). *Folia Anat. Jap., 14,* 15–45.

Holmdahl, D. E. 1939. Eine ganz junge (etwa 10 Tage alte) menschliche Embryonalanlage. *Upsala Läkareför. Förhandl., 45,* 363–371.

Hoyes, A. D. 1969. The human foetal yolk sac. An ultrastructural study of four specimens. *Z. Zellforsch., 99,* 469–490.

Iffy, L., Shepard, T. H., Jakobovits, A., Lemire, R. J., and Kerner, P. 1967. The rate of growth in young human embryos of Streeter's horizons XIII to XXIII. *Acta Anat., 66,* 178–186.

Ilieş, A. 1967. La topographie et la dynamique des zones nécrotiques normales chez l'embryon humain. I. *Rev. Roum. Embryol. Cytol., Sér. Embryol., 4,* 51–84.

Ingalls, N. W. 1918. A human embryo before the appearance of the myotomes. *Carnegie Inst. Wash. Publ. 227, Contrib. Embryol., 7,* 111–134.

Ingalls, N. W. 1920. A human embryo at the beginning of segmentation, with special reference to the vascular system. *Carnegie Inst. Wash. Publ. 274, Contrib. Embryol., 11,* 61–90.

Jacobson, A. G. 1966. Inductive processes in embryonic development. *Science, 152,* 25–34.

Jacobson, C. B., Sites, J. G., and Arias-Bernal, L. F. 1970. In vitro maturation and fertilization of human follicular oocytes. *Int. J. Fertil., 15,* 103–114.

Jahnke, V., and Stegner, H.-E. 1964. Ein menschlicher Keim von 15 bis 16 Tagen in situ. *Arch. Gynäkol., 200,* 88–98.

Jiménez Collado, J., and Ruano Gil, D. 1963. Descripcion de un embrion humano normal de 3 pares de somitos. *An. Desarrollo, 11,* 151–158.

Jirásek, J. E. 1971. *Development of the Genital System and Male Pseudohermaphroditism.* Johns Hopkins Press, Baltimore.

Jirásek, J. E., Uher, J., and Uhrová, M. 1966. Water and nitrogen content of the body of young human embryos. *Amer. J. Obstet. Gynecol.*, 96, 869–871.

Johnston, T. B. 1940. An early human embryo, with 0.55 mm. long embryonic shield. *J. Anat.*, London, 75, 1–49.

Johnston, T. B. 1941. The chorion and endometrium of the embryo H.R.1 *J. Anat.*, London, 75, 153–163.

Jones, H. O., and Brewer, J. I. 1941. A human embryo in the primitive-streak stage (Jones-Brewer ovum I). *Carnegie Inst. Wash. Publ. 525, Contrib. Embryol.*, 29, 157–165.

Jung, P. 1908. *Beiträge zur frühesten Ei-Einbettung beim menschlichen Weibe.* Karger, Berlin.

Kampmeier, C. F. 1929. On the problem of "parthenogenesis" in the mammalian ovary. *Amer. J. Anat.*, 43, 45–76.

Keibel, F. 1890. Ein sehr junges menschliches Ei. *Arch. Anat. Physiol.*, Anat. Abth., 250–267.

Keibel, [F.] 1907. Ueber ein junges, operativ gewonnenes menschliches Ei in situ. *Verh. Anat. Ges., Erg. Heft Anat. Anz.*, 30, 111–114.

Keibel, F., and Elze, C. 1908. *Normentafel zur Entwicklungsgeschichte des Menschen.* Fischer, Jena.

Keibel, F., and Mall, F. P. 1910 and 1912. *Manual of Human Embryology.* Volume 1 and Volume 2, Lippincott, Philadelphia.

Keller, R., and Keller, B. 1954. Implantation eines sehr jungen menschlichen Eies (wahrscheinlich weniger als 13 Tage alt) am äusseren Muttermund. *Zbl. Gynäkol.*, 76, 1–4.

Kennedy, J. F., and Donahue, R. P. 1969. Human oocytes: maturation in chemically defined media. *Science*, 164, 1292–1293.

Khvatov, B. P. 1967. Human embryo at the stage of blastodermic vesicle [in Russian]. *Arkh. Anat. Gistol. Embriol.*, 53, 51–56.

Khvatov, B. P. 1968. Phenomenon of parthenogenesis in atretic follicle of human ovary [in Russian]. *Arkh. Anat. Gistol. Embriol.*, 54, 93–96.

Kindred, J. E. 1933. A human embryo of the presomite period from the uterine tube. *Amer. J. Anat.*, 53, 221–241.

Kistner, R. W. 1953. A thirteen-day normal human embryo showing early villous and yolk-sac development. *Amer. J. Obstet. Gynecol.*, 65, 24–29.

Knorre, A. G. 1956. Cited by Mazanec (1959).

Kollmann, J. 1907. *Handatlas der Entwicklungsgeschichte des Menschen.* Vol. 1, Fischer, Jena.

Krafka, J. 1939. Parthenogenic cleavage in the human ovary. *Anat. Rec.*, 75, 19–21.

Krafka, J. 1941. The Torpin ovum, a presomite human embryo. *Carnegie Inst. Wash. Publ. 525, Contrib. Embryol.*, 29, 167–193.

Krafka, J. 1942. A free human tubal ovum in a late cleavage stage. *Anat. Rec.*, 82, 426.

Krause, W. 1953. Ein menschliches Ei mit 0.32 mm Keimschildlänge in Situ. *Z. Mikrosk.-Anat. Forsch.*, 59, 29–119.

Krukenberg. 1922. Ein junges menschliches Ei. *Zbl. Gynäkol.*, 46, 193–194.

Landesman, R. 1967. Neural-mesodermal interactions subsequent to neural induction in *Ambystoma. Develop. Biol.*, 16, 341–367.

Larsen, J. F. 1970. Electron miscroscopy of nidation in the rabbit and observations on the human trophoblastic invasion. In *Ovo-implantation. Human Gonadotropins and Prolactin.* Karger, Basel, pp. 38–51.

Lewis, B. V., and Harrison, R. G. 1966. A presomite human embryo showing a yolk-sac duct. *J. Anat.*, London, 100, 389–396.

Lewis, W. H., and Wright, E. S. 1935. On the early development of the mouse egg. *Carnegie Inst. Wash. Publ. 459, Contrib. Embryol.*, 25, 113–144.

Linzenmeier, G. 1914. Ein junges menschliches Ei in situ. *Arch. Gynäk.*, 102, 1–17.

Longo, F. J., and Anderson, E. 1969. Cytological events leading to the formation of the two-cell stage in the rabbit: association of the maternally and paternally derived genomes. *J. Ultrastruct. Res.*, 29, 86–118.

Lordy, C. 1931. A human ovum in its early phases of development. *Ann. Fac. Med. São Paulo*, 6, 29–35.

Luckett, W. P. 1971. The origin of extraembryonic mesoderm in the early human and rhesus monkey embryos. *Anat. Rec.*, 169, 369–370.

Luckett, W. P. 1973. Amniogenesis in the early human and rhesus monkey embryos. *Anat. Rec.*, 175, 375.

Ludwig, E. 1928. Über einen operativ gewonnenen menschlichen Embryo mit einem Ursegmente (Embryo Da 1). *Morph. Jahrb.*, 59, 41–104.

M'Intyre, D. 1926. The development of the vascular system in the human embryo prior to the establishment of the heart. *Trans. Roy. Soc. Edinburgh*, 55, 77–113.

McMurrich, J. P. 1930. *Leonardo da Vinci, the Anatomist, 1452–1519.* Williams and Wilkins, Baltimore.

REFERENCES

Mall, F. P. 1900. A contribution to the study of the pathology of early human embryos. *Johns Hopkins Hosp. Rep., 9,* 1–68.

Mall, F. P. 1907. On measuring human embryos. *Anat. Rec., 1,* 129–140.

Mall, F. P. 1913. A plea for an institute of human embryology. *J. Amer. Med. Ass., 60,* 1599–1601.

Mall, F. P. 1914. On stages in the development of human embryos from 2 to 25 mm. long. *Anat. Anz., 46,* 78–84.

Mall, F. P. 1916. The human magma réticulé in normal and in pathological development. *Carnegie Inst. Wash. Publ. 224, Contrib. Embryol., 4,* 5–26.

Mall, F. P., and Meyer, A. W. 1921. Studies on abortuses: a survey of pathologic ova in the Carnegie Embryological Collection. *Carnegie Inst. Wash. Publ. 275, Contrib. Embryol., 12,* 1–364.

Marchetti, A. A. 1945. A pre-villous human ovum accidentally recovered from a curettage specimen. *Carnegie Inst. Wash. Publ. 557, Contrib. Embryol., 31,* 107–115.

Martin, C. P., and Falkiner, N. McI. 1938. The Falkiner ovum. *Amer. J. Anat., 63,* 251–271.

Mazanec, K. 1953. *Blastogenesa člověka.* Státní Zdravotnické Nakladatelství, Prague.

Mazanec, K. 1959. *Blastogenese des Menschen.* Fischer, Jena.

Mazanec, K. 1960. A young human embryo "HEB-18" with a Hensen's node 0.071 mm long, before the Anlage of a head process. *Scripta Med., 33,* 185–194.

Mazanec, K., and Musilovà, M. 1959. A young human presomite embryo "HEB-42" with a headprocess 0.250 mm long (preliminary report). *Scripta Med., 32,* 261–270.

Menkin, M. F., and Rock, J. 1948. In vitro fertilization and cleavage of human ovarian eggs. *Amer. J. Obstet. Gynecol., 55,* 440–452.

Meyer, A. W. 1953. The elusive human allantois in older literature. In *Science, Medicine and History.* Oxford University Press, Oxford, pp. 510–520.

Meyer, P. 1924. Ein junges menschliches Ei mit 0,4 mm langem Embryonalschild. *Arch. Gynäk., 122,* 38–87.

Mintz, B. 1964. Formation of genetically mosaic mouse embryos, and early development of "lethal (t^{12}/t^{12})-normal" mosaics. *J. Exp. Zool., 157,* 273–291.

Moghissi, K. S., and Hafez, E. S. E. (ed.). 1972. *Biology of Mammalian Fertilization and Implantation.* Thomas, Springfield, Illinois.

von Möllendorff, W. 1921a. Über das jüngste bisher bekannte menschliche Abortivei (Ei Sch.). Ein Beitrag zur Lehre von der Einbettung des menschlichen Eies. *Z. Anat. Entwicklungsgesch., 62,* 352–405.

von Möllendorff, W. 1921b. Über einen jungen, operativ gewonnenen menschlichen Keim (Ei OP.). *Z. Anat. Entwicklungsges., 62,* 406–432.

von Möllendorff, W. 1925. Das menschliche Ei WO(lfring). Implantation, Verschluss der Implantationsöffnung und Keimesentwicklung beim Menschen vor Bildung des Primitivstreifens. *Z. Anat. Entwicklungsges., 76,* 16–42.

Morton, W. R. M. 1949. Two early human embryos. *J. Anat.,* London, *83,* 308–314.

Mossman, H. W. 1937. Comparative morphogenesis of the fetal membranes and accessory uterine structures. *Carnegie Inst. Wash. Publ. 479, Contrib. Embryol., 26,* 129–246.

Müller, S. 1930. Ein jüngstes menschliches Ei. *Z. Mikrosk.-Anat. Forsch., 20,* 175–184.

Mulnard, J. G. 1965. Studies of regulation of mouse ova *in vitro.* In G. E. W. Wolstenholme and M. O'Connor (ed.), *Preimplantation Stages of Pregnancy* (Ciba Foundation Symposium). Churchill, London, pp. 123–144.

Mulnard, J. G. 1967. Analyse microcinématographique du développement de l'oeuf de souris du stade II au blastocyste. *Arch. Biol.,* Liège, *78,* 107–139.

Nicolet, G. 1970a. Analyse autoradiographique de la localisation des différentes ébauches présomptives dans la ligne primitive de l'embryon de Poulet. *J. Embryol. Exp. Morphol., 23,* 79–108.

Nicolet, G. 1970b. Is the presumptive notochord responsible for somite genesis in the chick? *J. Embryol. Exp. Morphol., 24,* 467–478.

Nishimura, H., Takano, K., Tanimura, T., and Yasuda, M. 1968. Normal and abnormal development of human embryos. *Teratol., 1,* 281–290.

Noback, C. R., Paff, G. H., and Poppiti, R. J. 1968. A bilaminar human ovum. *Acta. Anat., 69,* 485–496.

Noyes, R. W., Dickmann, Z., Clewe, T. H., and Bonney, W. A. 1965. Pronuclear ovum from a patient using an intrauterine contraceptive device. *Science, 147,* 744–745.

Odgers, P. N. B. 1937. An early human ovum (Thomson) *in situ. J. Anat.,* London, *71,* 161–168.

Odgers, P. N. B. 1941. A presomite human embryo with a neurenteric canal (embryo R. S.). *J. Anat.,* London, *75,* 381–388.

van Oordt, G. J. 1921. Early developmental stages of Manis javanica Desm. *Verh. Konink. Akad. Wetensch. Amsterdam, 21,* pp. 102.

O'Rahilly, R. 1963. The early development of the otic vesicle in staged human embryos. *J. Embryol. Exp. Morphol., 11,* 741–755.

O'Rahilly, R. 1970. The manifestation of the axes of the human embryo. *Z. Anat. Entwicklungsgesch., 132,* 50–57.

O'Rahilly, R. 1971. The timing and sequence of events in human cardiogenesis. *Acta Anat., 79,* 70–75.

O'Rahilly, R., and Gardner, E. 1971. The timing and sequence of events in the development of the human nervous system during the embryonic period proper. *Z. Anat. Entwicklungsgesch., 134,* 1–12.

Orts Llorca, F., Jiménez Collado, J., and Ruano Gil, D. 1960. La fase plexiforme del desarrollo cardiaco en el hombre. Embriones de 21 ± 1 dia. *An. Desarrollo, 8,* 79–98.

Padget, D. H. 1970. Neuroschisis and human embryonic maldevelopment. New evidence on anencephaly, spina bifida and diverse mammalian defects. *J. Neuropathol. Exp. Neurol., 29,* 192–216.

Park, W. W. 1957. The occurrence of sex chromatin in early human and macaque embryos. *J. Anat., London, 91,* 369–373.

Pasteels, J. 1940. Un aperçu comparatif de la gastrulation chez les Chordés. *Biol. Rev., 15,* 59–106.

Pasteels, J. 1945. On the formation of the primary entoderm of the duck (Anas domestica) and on the significance of the bilaminar embryo in birds. *Anat. Rec., 93,* 5–21.

Patten, B. M., and Philpott, R. 1921. The shrinkage of embryos in the processes preparatory to sectioning. *Anat. Rec., 20,* 393–413.

Penkert. 1910. Über ein sehr junges Ei in der Tube. *Zbl. Gynäk., 34,* 345–347.

Peters, H. 1899. *Über die Einbettung des menschlichen Eies und das früheste bisher bekannte menschliche Placentationsstadium.* Deuticke, Leipzig.

Petrov, G. N. 1958. Fertilization and the first cleavage stages in the human ovum outside the organism [in Russian]. *Arkh. Anat. Gistol. Embriol., 35,* 88–91.

Piersol, W. H. 1937. A human embryo of two somites, in situ. *Anat. Rec., 67 suppl.,* 39–40.

Politzer, G. 1933. Die Keimbahn des Menschen. *Z. Anat. Entwicklungsgesch., 100,* 331–361.

Pommerenke, W. T. 1958. A twelfth night ovum. *Fertil. Steril., 9,* 400–406.

Potts, D. M. 1968. The ultrastructure of implantation in the mouse. *J. Anat., London, 103,* 77–90.

Potts, D. M., and Wilson, I. B. 1967. The preimplantation conceptus of the mouse at 90 hours *post coitum. J. Anat., London, 102,* 1–11.

Ramsey, E. M. 1937. The Lockyer embryo: an early human embryo *in situ. Carnegie Inst. Wash. Publ. 479, Contrib. Embryol., 26,* 99–120.

Ramsey, E. M. 1938. The Yale embryo. *Carnegie Inst. Wash. Publ. 496, Contrib. Embryol., 27,* 67–84.

Reinius, S. 1967. Ultrastructure of blastocyst attachment in the mouse. *Z. Zellforsch., 77,* 257–266.

Reynolds, S. R. M. 1954. Developmental changes and future requirements. *In* The Mammalian Fetus: Physiological Aspects of Development. *Cold Spring Harbor Symp. Quant. Biol., 19,* 1–2.

Richter, K. M. 1952. A new human embryo having an estimated age of fifteen days. *Anat. Rec., 112,* 462.

Robertson, G. G., O'Neill, S. L., and Chappell, R. H. 1948. On a normal human embryo of 17 days development. *Anat. Rec., 100,* 9–28.

Rock, J., and Hertig, A. T. 1941. Two human ova of the pre-villous stage, having an ovulation age of about eleven and twelve days respectively. *Carnegie Inst. Wash. Publ., 525, Contrib. Embryol., 29,* 127–156.

Rock, J., and Hertig, A. T. 1942. Some aspects of early human development. *Amer. J. Obstet. Gynecol., 44,* 973–983.

Rock, J., and Hertig, A. T. 1944. Information regarding the time of human ovulation derived from a study of 3 unfertilized and 11 fertilized ova. *Amer. J. Obstet. Gynecol., 47,* 343–356.

Rock, J., and Hertig, A. T. 1945. Two human ova of the pre-villous stage, having a developmental age of about seven and nine days respectively. *Carnegie Inst. Wash. Publ. 557, Contrib. Embryol., 31,* 65–84.

Rock, J., and Hertig, A. T. 1948. The human conceptus during the first two weeks of gestation. *Amer. J. Obstet. Gynecol., 55,* 6–17.

Rock, J., and Hertig, A. T. 1949. Two human ova of the pre-villous stage, having a developmental age of about 8 and 9 days respectively. *Carnegie Inst. Wash. Publ. 583, Contrib. Embryol., 33,* 169–186.

Rosenquist, G. C. 1966. A radioautographic study of labeled grafts in the chick blastoderm. Development from primitive-streak stages to stage 12. *Carnegie Inst. Wash. Publ. 625, Contrib. Embryol., 38,* 71–110.

Rossenbeck, H. 1923. Ein junges menschliches Ei. Ovum humanum Peh. 1-Hochstetter. *Z. Anat. Entwicklungsgesch., 68,* 325–385.

Schlafke, S., and Enders, A. C. 1967. Cytological changes during cleavage and blastocyst formation in the rat. *J. Anat.*, London, *102*, 13–32.

Schlagenhaufer, [F.], and Verocay, [F.] 1916. Ein junges menschliches Ei. *Arch. Gynäkol.*, *105*, 151–168.

Scipiades, E. 1938. Young human ovum detected in uterine scraping. *Carnegie Inst. Wash. Publ. 496, Contrib. Embryol.*, *27*, 95–105.

Severn, C. B. 1971. A morphological study of the development of the human liver. I. Development of the hepatic diverticulum. *Amer. J. Anat.*, *131*, 133–158.

Shaw, W. 1932. Observations on two specimens of early human ova. *Brit. Med. J.*, *1*, 411–415.

Shettles, L. B. 1956. A morula stage of human ovum developed in vitro. *Clin. Excerpts, 18*, 92–93.

Shettles, L. B. 1957. Parthenogenetic cleavage of the human ovum. *Bull. Sloane Hosp. Women, 3*, 59–61.

Shettles, L. B. 1958. The living human ovum. *Amer. J. Obstet. Gynecol.*, *76*, 398–406.

Shettles, L. B. 1960. *Ovum Humanum*. Hafner, New York.

Smith, D. W. 1970. *Recognizable Patterns of Human Malformation. Genetic, Embryologic, and Clinical Aspects*. Saunders, Philadelphia.

von Spee, F. 1896. Neue Beobachtungen über sehr frühe Entwicklungsstufen des menschlichen Eies. *Arch. Anat. Physiol., Anat. Abth.*, 1–30.

Springer, M. 1972. Der Canalis neurentericus beim Menschen. *Z. Kinderchir.*, *11*, 183–189 and 192–194.

Starck, D. 1956. Die Frühphase der menschlichen Embryonalentwicklung und ihre Bedeutung für die Beurteilung der Säugerontogenese. *Ergeb. Anat. Entwicklungsgesch.*, *35*, 133–175.

Steptoe, P. C., Edwards, R. G., and Purdy, J. M. 1971. Human blastocysts grown in culture. *Nature, 229*, 132–133.

Stewart, H. L. 1952. Duration of pregnancy and postmaturity. *J. Amer. Med. Ass.*, *148*, 1079–1083.

Stieve, H. 1926. Ein 13 ½-Tage altes, in der Gebärmutter erhaltenes und durch Eingriff gewonnenes menschliches Ei. *Z. Mikrosk.-Anat. Forsch.*, *7*, 295–402.

Stieve, H. 1931. Die Dottersackbildung beim Ei des Menschen. *Anat. Anz., 72*, 44–56.

Stieve, H. 1936. Ein ganz junges, in der Gebärmutter erhaltenes menschliches Ei (Keimling Werner). *Z. Mikrosk.-Anat. Forsch.*, *40*, 281–322.

Strahl, H. 1916. Über einen jungen menschlichen Embryo nebst Bemerkungen zu C. Rabl's Gastrulationstheorie. *Anat. Hefte, 54*, 113–147.

Strauss, F. 1945. Gedanken zur Entwicklung des Amnions und des Dottersackes beim Menschen. *Rev. Suisse Zool.*, *52*, 213–229.

Streeter, G. L. 1920. A human embryo (Mateer) of the presomite period. *Carnegie Inst. Wash. Publ. 272, Contrib. Embryol.*, *9*, 389–424.

Streeter, G. L. 1920. Weight, sitting height, head size, foot length and menstrual age of the human embryo. *Carnegie Inst. Wash. Publ. 274, Contrib. Embryol.*, *11*, 143–170.

Streeter, G. L. 1926. The "Miller" ovum—the youngest normal human embryo thus far known. *Carnegie Inst. Wash. Publ. 363, Contrib. Embryol.*, *18*, 31–48.

Streeter, G. L. 1927. Development of the mesoblast and notochord in pig embryos. *Carnegie Inst. Wash. Publ. 380, Contrib. Embryol.*, *19*, 73–92.

Streeter, G. L. 1937. Origin of the yolk sac in primates. *Anat. Rec., 70* suppl., 53–54.

Streeter, G. L. 1939a. A new profile reconstruction of the Miller ovum. *Anat. Rec., 73* suppl., 75.

Streeter, G. L. 1939b. New reconstruction of the Miller ovum. *Carnegie Inst. Wash. Year Book 38*, 149.

Streeter, G. L. 1942. Developmental horizons in human embryos. Description of age group XI, 13 to 20 somites, and age group XII, 21 to 29 somites. *Carnegie Inst. Wash. Publ. 541, Contrib. Embryol.*, *30*, 211–245.

Streeter, G. L. 1945. Developmental horizons in human embryos. Description of age group XIII, embryos about 4 or 5 millimeters long, and age group XIV, period of indentation of the lens vesicle. *Carnegie Inst. Wash. Publ. 557, Contrib. Embryol.*, *31*, 27–63.

Streeter, G. L. 1948. Developmental horizons in human embryos. Description of age groups XV, XVI, XVII, and XVIII, being the third issue of a survey of the Carnegie Collection. *Carnegie Inst. Wash. Publ. 575, Contrib. Embryol.*, *32*, 133–203.

Streeter, G. L. 1951. Developmental horizons in human embryos. Description of age groups XIX, XX, XXI, XXII, and XXIII, being the fifth issue of a survey of the Carnegie Collection. *Carnegie Inst. Wash. Publ. 592, Contrib. Embryol.*, *34*, 165–196.

Studnička, F. K. 1929. Über den Zusammenhang des Cytoplasmas bei jungen menschlichen Embryonen. *Z. Mikrosk.-Anat. Forsch.*, *18*, 553–656.

Studnička, F. K., and Florian, J. 1928. Les cytodesmes et le mésostroma chez quelques jeunes embryons humains. *C. R. Ass. Anat.*, 23, 437–443.

Stump, C. W. 1929. A human blastocyst *in situ*. *Trans. Roy. Soc. Edinburgh*, 56, 191–202.

Tao, T.-W., and Hertig, A. T. 1965. Viability and differentiation of human trophoblast in organ culture. *Amer. J. Anat.*, 116, 315–327.

Tarkowski, A. J. 1965a. Discussion of paper by Mulnard. See Mulnard (1965).

Tarkowski, A. J. 1965b. Embryonic and postnatal development of mouse chimeras. In G. E. W. Wolstenholme and M. O'Connor (ed.), *Preimplantation Stages of Pregnancy* (Ciba Foundation Symposium). Churchill, London, pp. 183–193.

Teacher, J. H. 1925. On the implantation of the human ovum and the early development of the trophoblast. *Z. Anat. Entwicklungsgesch.*, 76, 360–385.

Thibault, C. 1967. Analyse comparée de la fécondation et de ses anomalies chez la brebis, la vache et la lapine. *Ann. Biol. Animale Biochem. Biophys.*, 7, 5–23.

Thomas, F., and van Campenhout, E. 1953. Étude d'un oeuf humain d'approximativement 17 jours. Découverte d'autopsie médicolégale. *Ann. Méd. Légale*, Paris, 33, 193–199.

Thomas, F., and van Campenhout, E. 1963. Untersuchung eines, bei einer gerichtlichen Sektion nachgewiesenen, etwa 11 Tage alten menschlichen Eies. *Deutsche Z. Gerichtl. Med.*, 54, 119–123.

Thompson, P., and Brash, J. C. 1923. A human embryo with head-process and commencing archenteric canal. *J. Anat.*, London, 58, 1–20.

Toivonen, S., and Saxén, L. 1968. Morphogenetic interaction of presumptive neural and mesodermal cells mixed in different ratios. *Science*, 159, 539–540.

Treloar, A. E., Behn, G. B., and Cowan, D. W. 1967. Analysis of gestational interval. *Amer. J. Obstet. Gynecol.*, 99, 34–45.

Triepel, H. 1916. Ein menschlicher Embryo mit Canalis neurentericus. Chordulation. *Anat. Hefte*, 54, 149–185.

Turner, C. L. 1920. A wax model of a presomite human embryo. *Anat. Rec.*, 19, 372–412.

Vaage, S. 1969. The segmentation of the primitive neural tube in chick embryos (Gallus domesticus). A morphological, histochemical and autoradiographical investigation. *Ergeb. Anat. Entwicklungsgesch.*, 41, 1–88.

Vakaet, L. 1960. Quelques précisions sur la cinématique de la ligne primitive chez le Poulet. *J. Embryol. Exp. Morphol.*, 8, 321–326.

Vakaet, L. 1971. Échanges de fragments d'ectophylle de caille et de poulet. *C. R. Ass. Anat.*, 56, 770–777.

Van Beneden, E. 1899. Sur la présence, chez l'homme, d'un canal archentérique. *Anat. Anz.*, 15, 349–356.

di Virgilio, G., Lavenda, N., and Worden, J. L. 1967. Sequence of events in neural tube closure and the formation of neural crest in the chick embryo. *Acta Anat.*, 68, 127–146.

Vollman, R. F. 1967. The length of the premenstrual phase by age of women. *Proc. 5th World Congr. Fertil. Steril.*, Stockholm (1966), Excerpta Med. Internat. Congr. Series, No. 113, 1171–1175.

Waldeyer, A. 1929a. Ein junges menschliches Ei in situ [Schö(nholz)]. *Z. Anat. Entwicklungsgesch.*, 90, 412–457.

Waldeyer, A. 1929b. Mesodermbildung bei einem jungen menschlichen Embryo. *Anat. Anz.*, 35, 145–151.

West, C. M. 1952. Two presomite human embryos. *J. Obstet. Gynaecol. Brit. Emp.*, 59, 336–351.

Wilder, H. H. 1904. Duplicate twins and double monsters. *Amer. J. Anat.*, 3, 387–472.

Wilens, S. (ed.). 1969. *R. G. Harrison: Organization and Development of the Embryo*. Yale Univ. Press, New Haven, Connecticut.

Willis, R. A. 1962. *The Borderland of Embryology and Pathology*. 2nd edition, Butterworths, London.

Wilson, J. T. 1914. Observations upon young human embryos. *J. Anat.*, London, 48, 315–351.

Wilson, K. M. 1945. A normal human ovum of sixteen days development (the Rochester ovum). *Carnegie Inst. Wash. Publ.* 557, Contrib. Embryol., 31, 101–106.

Wilson, K. M. 1954. A previllous ovum of eleven days development. *Amer. J. Obstet. Gynecol.*, 68, 63–68.

Witschi, E. 1956a. *Development of Vertebrates*. Saunders, Philadelphia.

Witschi, E. 1956b. Proposals for an international agreement on normal stages in vertebrate embryology. *Proc. 14th Internat. Congr. Zool.*, Copenhagen (1953), pp. 260–262.

Witschi, E. 1962. Prenatal vertebrate development. In P. L. Altman and D. S. Dittmer (ed.), *Growth* (Biological Handbook). Federation Amer. Soc. Exp. Biol., Washington, D. C.

Young, M. P., Whicher, J. T., and Potts, D. M. 1968. The ultrastructure of implantation in

REFERENCES

the golden hamster *(Cricetus auratus).* J. Embryol. Exp. Morphol., 19, 341–345.

Zamboni, L. 1971. *Fine Morphology of Mammalian Fertilization.* Harper and Row, New York.

Zamboni, L. 1972. Fertilization in the mouse. In Moghissi, K. S., and Hafez, E. S. E. (ed.). *Biology of Mammalian Fertilization and Implantation.* Ch. 8 (pp. 213–262).

Zamboni, L., Mishell, D. R., Bell, J. H., and Baca, M. 1966. Fine structure of the human ovum in the pronuclear stage. J. Cell Biol., 30, 579–600.

SPECIMEN INDEX

The following is an alphabetical list of named and numbered specimens that have been described or cited in the literature. Their authors have also been included in the list. In the case of each specimen, the stage to which it is believed to belong is indicated, and further details will be found in the text under the heading of the appropriate stage.

Specimen or Author	Stage	Specimen or Author	Stage
Am. 10	6b	7850 (path.)	5–6
Andô	6b	7950	5c
D'Arrigo, 1961	7?	8000 (path.)	5c
		8004	5b
Bagiński and Borsuk, 1967	9	8020	5a
Bandler, 1912	5	8139	5c
Barnes	5c	8155	5a
Bayer	6b	8171	5b
Beitler (No. 763)	8?	8190 (path.)	2
Beneke	6b	8215	5b
Bi I	6b	8225	5a
Bi 24	7	8260	2
Biggart	7(6?)	8290 (path.)	6?
Boerner-Patzelt and Schwarzacher, 1923	8	8299 (path.)	5c
		8329 (path.)	5c
		8330	5c
Brewer, 1937, 1938 (Edwards-Jones-Brewer)	6b	8360	6a
		8370 (path.)	5c
Broman, 1936	8	8450 (path.)	2
Bryce, 1924 (M'Intyre)	8	8452 (path.)	2
(Teacher-Bryce I)	5	8500.1	2
(Teacher-Bryce II)	6b	8558	5c
		8602	7
Carnegie No. 763	8?	8630 (path.)	2
1399	7	8663	3
1878	9	8671	8
4900	5c	8672	6a
5080	9	8698	2
5960	8	8727	8
5981	8	8794	3
5982	9	8819	6b
6026 (path.)	6b?	8820	8
6027	8?	8904	2
6630	8	8905	6
6706	6–8?	9009	8
6734	6a	9350	5b
6815	8		
6900	6a	Da 1 (No. 5982)	9
7634	6a	Dankmeijer and Wielenga, 1968	5
7640	8	D'Arrigo, 1971	7?
7699	5c	Davies, 1944 (Davies-Harding)	5c
7700	5c	Debeyre, 1912	7
7762	6b	Dible-West, 1941	5c
7770 (path.)	5c	Dickmann et al., 1965	1
7771 (path.)	5c	Dobbin	8
7800 (path.)	7	Doyle et al., 1966	2
7801	6b	Dy	8
7802	7		

Specimen or Author	Stage
E.B.	6a
Edwards and Fowler, 1970	2, 3
Edwards et al., 1966	2
1969	1
1970	2
Edwards-Jones-Brewer (No. 8819)	6b
Eternod, 1899, 1909 (Vulliet)	8
Faber, 1940 (E.B.)	6a
Fahrenholz, 1927 (Ho)	7
Falkiner	7
Fetzer, 1910	6b
Fife-Richter	6b
Fitzgerald	7
Fitzgerald-Brewer I	8
II	7
Florian. See Bi I, Manchester 1285, T.F., etc.	
Frassi, 1908	8
Fruhling et al., 1954	5a
Gar	7
George, 1942 (No. 7640)	8
Gladstone and Hamilton, 1941 (Shaw)	8
Gläveke	8
Gle. See Gläveke	
Goodwin	7
Graf Spee (Gläveke)	8
Greenhill, 1927	6?
Grosser, 1913 (Kl. 13)	8
1922 (Kleinhans)	5c
1931 (H. Schm. 10)	7
1931 (Wa 17)	8
Guá	7(8?)
Gv (Madrid)	9
H3	9
H381	6
H.R. 1	6b(8?)
H. Schm. 10	7
Häggström, 1922	2
Hamilton. 1946, 1949	1
Hamilton and Boyd. 1960 (Missen)	7
Hamilton et al., 1943 (Barnes)	5c
1967	6?
Harrison and Jeffcoate, 1953 (Liverpool I)	6b
Harvard No. 55	6a
825	6b
HEB-18	6b
HEB-37	7
HEB-42	8
Herranz and Vásquez, 1964	2
Hertig and Rock. See specimen numbers under Carnegie	8
Hertig et al., 1958 ("No. 55")	6a
Herzog, 1909 (Manila)	6
Heuser, 1932 (No. 5960)	8
1954 (No. 9009)	8

Specimen or Author	Stage
Heuser. See also specimen numbers under Carnegie	
Hill. See Bi 24, Dobbin, etc.	
Hiramatsu, 1936 (Andô)	6b
His embryo E	9–10
Ho	7
Hugo	7
Ingalls, 1918 (Western Reserve No. 1)	8
1920 (No. 1878)	9
Jahnke and Stegner, 1964	6
Jiménez Collado and Ruano Gil (Gv)	9
Johnston, 1940 (H.R.1)	6b(8?)
Johnstone, 1914	6
Jones-Brewer I, 1941 (No. 8820)	8
II	7
Jung, 1908	6
Keibel, 1890 (Bayer)	6b
1907 (Frassi)	8
Keller and Keller, 1954	5
Khvatov, 1959	1
1967	3
1968	2
Kindred, 1933 (Goodwin)	7
Kistner, 1953	6
Kl. 13	8
Kleinhans	5c
Knorre (VMA-1)	6a
Krafka, 1939	2
1941 (Torpin)	6a
1942	3(2?)
Krause, 1953 (Am. 10)	6b
Krukenberg, 1922	8
Lbg	6b
Lewis and Harrison, 1966 (Liverpool II)	6b
Linzenmeier, 1914 (Stöckel)	6a
Liverpool I	6b
Liverpool II	6b
Lockyer (No. 6026)	6b?
Lordy, 1931 (Guá)	7(8?)
Lqt	8
Ludwig, 1928 (Da 1)	9
Macafee	5
M'Intyre, 1926	8
Mal	7
Manchester No. 1285	7
Manila	6
Marchetti, 1945 (No. 8139)	5c
Martin and Falkiner, 1938	7
Mateer (No. 1399)	7
Mazanec, 1960 (HEB-18)	6b
Mazanec and Musilovà, 1959 (HEB-42)	8

SPECIMEN INDEX

Specimen or Author	Stage
Menkin and Rock, 1948	
(No. 8260)	2
(No. 8500.1)	2
Merrill	6
Meyer, 1924 (P.M.)	7
Miller (No. 4900)	5c
Minot (Harvard No. 825)	6b
Missen	7
v. Möllendorff. See Von Möllendorff	
Morton, 1949 (Biggart)	7(6?)
(Macafee)	5
Müller, 1930	5
Noback et al., 1968	6
Normentafel 1 (Frassi)	8
2 (Gläveke)	8
Noyes et al., 1965	1
Odgers, 1937 (Thomson)	6b
1941 (R.S.)	8
Op	6b
P.M.	7
Peh.1-Hochstetter	8
Penkert, 1910	6b?
Peters, 1899	6a
Petrov, 1968	2
Pha I	7
Pha II	7
Pha XVII	8
Piersol, 1937 (T439)	9
Pommerenke, 1958	5
R.S.	8
Ramsey, 1937 (Lockyer)	6b?
1938 (Yale)	6a
Richter, 1952 (Fife-Richter)	6b
Robertson et al., 1948	7(8?)
Rochester (No. 7762)	6b
Rossenbeck, 1923 (Peh.1-Hochstetter)	8
Sch	5
Schlagenhaufer and Verocay, 1916	6
Schö	8
Scipiades, 1938	5(6?)
Shaw	3
Shettles, 1956, 1957, 1960	
1958, 1960, 1969	2

Specimen or Author	Stage
Stieve, 1926 (Hugo)	7
1936 (Werner)	5c
Stöckel (No. 6900)	6a
Strahl, 1916	8
Strahl-Beneke	6b
Streeter, 1920 (Mateer)	7
1926 (Miller)	5c
Stump, 1929 (H381)	6
Swett (No. 6815)	8
T439 (Toronto)	9
T.F.	6b
Teacher-Bryce I	5
Teacher-Bryce II	6b
Thomas and van Campenhout, 1953	6
1963	5?
Thompson and Brash, 1923	8
Thomson	6b
Thyng (No. 6026)	6b?
Torpin (No. 7634)	6a
Triepel, 1916 (Dy)	8
v. H. (von Herff)	6
VMA-1 (Knorre)	6a
Von Möllendorff, 1921 (Op)	6b
1921 (Sch.)	5
1925 (Wo)	6b
Von Spee, 1889, 1896 (Gläveke)	8
1896 (v. H.)	6
Vuill. See Vulliet	
Vulliet	8
Wa17	8
Waldeyer, 1929 (Schö)	8
Way and Dawson, 1959	2
Werner	5c
West, 1952 (Gar)	7
1952 (Mal)	7
Western Reserve No. 1	8
Wharton (No. 6706)	6–8?
Wilson, 1914 (H3)	9
1945 (Rochester)	6b
1954	5c
Wo	6b
Yale (No. 6734)	6a
Zamboni et al., 1966	1

INDEX

Note: Entries are listed here under nouns (e.g., disc) rather than under descriptive adjectives (e.g., embryonic).

Age, embryonic, 5
  postovulatory, 5, 9
Allantois, 69, 92, 129
Amniogenesis, 30, 39, 43, 44, 51
Amnion, 38, 39, 44, 51, 64, 83, 104
Angiogenesis, 50, 64, 88
Aortae, dorsal, 128
Arches, aortic, 128
Area, mesodermal proliferating, 50, 64, 80
  protocardiac, 87
  trigeminal nerve, 126
Arteries, internal carotid, 128
  umbilical, 110, 129
Axialization, 68

Bauchstiel, 53
Blastocoel, 23
Blastocyst, 23, 29
Blastodisc, 64
Blastopore, 66
Blastula, 23
Body, polar, 10
Born reconstructions, 1
Brain, 125
Branchial, 126

Canal, chordal, 106
  Lieberkühn's, 81, 94, 95, 106
  neurenteric, 103, 106, 129
  notochordal, 86, 103, 106
Cavity, amniotic, 38, 44, 51, 64
  blastocyst, 24
  chorionic, 33
  pericardial, 106, 127
  segmentation, 23, 24
Cells, formative, 23
  primordial germ, 25, 28, 53, 66, 69, 72, 81, 92, 95, 102, 105, 113
Chordafortsatzkanal, 106
Chordamesoderm, 105
Chorion, 33, 45, 47, 59, 83
Chromatin, sex, 26, 50, 63, 89, 104
Circle, lacunar vascular, 47
Cleavage, 11, 15, 23, 24
Clefts, pharyngeal, 126
Closing-plug, 47
Clumps, cytotrophoblastic, 44, 50, 62
Coelom, 127
  pericardial, 106, 127
Collection, Carnegie, 1
Columns, cytotrophoblastic, 62
Complex, prochordal, 107

Corona radiata, 10
C.-R. length, 4
Crest, mesoblastic, 50, 62
  neural, 105, 125
Cytodesmata, 66, 106
Cytotrophoblast, 30, 33, 35, 50, 62

Death, cell, 67, 105
Decidua, 33, 47, 59, 83, 104
  basalis, 59
  capsularis, 59, 104
  parietalis, 59, 104
Decidualization, 29
Delamination, 37
Dextrocardia, 138
Differentiation, axial, 59, 68
Disc, embryonic, 39, 44, 51, 64, 66, 68, 104
  germ, 23
  otic, 125
Diverticulum, allanto-enteric, 70, 89, 110, 129
  allantoic, 69, 89, 110, 129
  yolk sac, 69, 70, 88, 110, 129
Dorsalization, 26
Dorsoventrality, 26
Dotterpropf, 105
Dottersackanlage, 45
Duct, amniotic, 64, 73, 86, 123
  yolk sac, 73

Ectoderm, amniotic, 64, 66, 83
  embryonic, 66, 105
Embryonalanlage, 64
Embryonalschild, 64
Endknoten, 86
Endocardium, 106, 121, 128
Endoderm, 23, 26, 39, 51, 66, 105
Endometrium, 35, 43, 47
Entwicklungsreihe, 2
Epiblast, 23, 39, 44, 51, 66
Epimyocardium, 128
Ergänzungsplatte, 107
Erythroblasts, primitive, 89, 112

Features, axial, 59
Fertilization, 9
Flexure, cranial, 125
  mesencephalic, 125
Fold, caudal, 125
  head, 125
  neural, 125
Forebrain, 125
Foregut, 110, 126

Gastrulation, 126
Gewebspilz, 47
Groove, medullary, 105
  neural, 105, 125
  primitive, 67, 86, 110
Gut, 126

Heart, 106, 121
Height, sitting, 4
Hematopoiesis, 69, 89
Hemocytoblasts, 89, 110
Heukelom, S. van, 62
Hindbrain, 125
Hindgut, 110, 126
His, W., 1
Horizons, developmental, 2

Implantation, 29, 33
Interval, gestational, 9
Islands, blood, 64, 89, 92, 110, 129

Jelly, cardiac, 128
Junction, fetal-maternal, 62

Keibel, F., 1
Keimanlage, 64
Keimling, 64
Keimscheibe, 64
Knot, Hensen's, 67, 86
Kopffortsatz, 87
Kopffortsatzkanal, 106

Lacunae, 43, 44, 50
Langhans, T., 63
Layer, Langhans', 63
Length, C.-R., 4
Leonardo da Vinci, 4

Mall, F. P., 1, 2
Mass, inner cell, 17, 23, 25, 30
Mazanec's groups, 7
Membrana prima, 66, 72
Membrane, buccopharyngeal, 125, 127
  cloacal, 69, 89, 110, 129
  exocoelomic, 44, 45, 51, 69
  oropharyngeal, 125, 127
Mesoblast, embryonic, 68, 86, 105, 127
  extra-embryonic, 37, 50, 63
Mesocardium, 128
Mesoderm, 127
  intermediate, 127
  paraxial, 127
Midbrain, 125
Morula, 15
Myocardium, 128
Myocoele, 121, 127

Necrosis, cellular, 67, 105
Neuromeres, 125
Node, end, 70, 86
  primitive, 67, 86, 105
Normality, 8

Normentafeln, 2
Notch, terminal, 125
Notochord, 88

Occlusion-plug, 47
Oocyte, 9
  penetrated, 10
Ootid, 10
Operculum, 47
Organizer, 105
Ovum, 9

Parthenogenesis, 17, 18, 26
Pit, primitive, 103, 106
Placenta, 43, 83
Plate, alar, 105
  basal, 105
  cardiogenic, 128
  closing, 47
  completion, 107
  lateral, 127
  neural, 104
  notochordal, 106, 128
  otic, 125
  prechordal, 68, 88, 106, 129
  prochordal, 107
  protochordal, 107
Plasmodium, 30
Plexus, endocardial, 106, 121, 128
  vitelline, 129
Plug, closing, 47
  occlusion, 47
Portal, intestinal, 126
Pouches, pharyngeal, 126
Praechordalplatte, 107
Process, head, 87
  notochordal, 83, 87, 88, 106
Prolongement céphalique, 87
Proneuromeres, 125
Pronuclei, 9, 11
Pseudomorula, 24
Pseudoparthenogenesis, 17

Reaction, decidual, 44, 47, 59, 83
  predecidual, 44, 47
  stromal, 44
Reconstructions, 1
Rhombomeres, 125
Riesenform, 104
Rudiment, embryonic, 64

Sac, yolk, 44, 45, 51, 69, 88, 110, 129
Schizolig, 15
Schlusscoagulum, 47
Septum transversum, 128
Seriation, embryological, 1
Shell, cytotrophoblastic, 62, 83
Shield, embryonic, 39, 64
Sichelknoten, 86
Situs inversus viscerum, 138
Somites, 123, 127

INDEX

Space, intervillous, 59, 83
   perivitelline, 10
   subzonal, 10
Specificity, human, 9
Stages, embryonic, 2, 3, 7
   pre-implantation, 123
   presomite, 123
   previllous, 123
   somite, 123
Stalk, amnio-embryonic, 70
   connecting, 53, 70, 110, 129
   umbilical, 70
Stems, primary villous, 62, 83
Stomodeum, 127
Streak, primitive, 66, 86, 105, 127
Streeter, G. L., 2
Sulci of heart, 128
Symmetry, bilateral, 68
Symplasma, 31, 37
Syncytiotrophoblast, 30, 33, 36, 44, 50, 62
Syncytium, 30, 37

Trophoblast, 17, 23, 33, 35, 44
Twins, conjoined, 33, 122
   dizygotic, 17
   monozygotic, 15, 23, 33, 82, 122

Veins, omphalomesenteric, 128
   umbilical, 110, 129
Verschlusspfropf, 47
Vesicle, exocoelomic, 44
Vessels, blood, 50, 64, 70, 127
   umbilical, 70, 110
Villi, chorionic, 59, 62, 83

Weight, body, 5
Witschi's stages, 7

Zona pellucida, 9, 25, 29
Zone, annular, 69, 107
   border, 62
   penetration, 62
Zwergform, 104
Zygote, 11